Little Giants

Nutritious Eating for Mighty Kids

by

Sarah Parker

Table of Contents

Introduction

Welcome to a journey that embarks upon the delightful yet intricate world of nurturing healthy eating habits in children. As parents, caregivers, educators, and healthcare professionals, you are the frontline advocates, mentors, and enablers of the next generation's dietary patterns. Your impact on their lives extends beyond the immediate; it shapes their relationship with food, their health, and ultimately, their happiness.

Instilling a love for wholesome food and balanced meals in kids can be like navigating a ship through uncharted waters. It's a voyage filled with the joys of discovery, the challenges of unanticipated obstacles, and the satisfaction of watching children thrive. The goal of this book is clear and compelling: to empower you with the comprehensive knowledge and practical tools needed to guide children towards a dietary lifestyle that will support their growth and foster their well-being.

Let's start with understanding the building blocks of good nutrition. The foundations laid during childhood can last a lifetime, making an insightful overview of macronutrients and micronutrients critical. However, we won't dive deep into these topics right now—that's what awaits you in the coming chapters.

We'll navigate the principles of creating a positive food environment and the benefit of establishing consistent eating routines. There's a subtle art to balancing what's on a child's plate, which can sometimes feel more like complex choreography than simply meal planning. And this doesn't just involve the food itself but also the patterns and socializations formed around eating.

With patience and creativity, even the pickiest of eaters can join the clean plate club. It's all about understanding their unique challenges and finding smart, individual solutions. As we venture through the pages, you'll find tips and anecdotes tailored for handling everything from a hectic family schedule to the child who simply says "no" to greens.

The role you play cannot be overstated. Your everyday choices, responses to food, and mealtime discussions have a profound influence on developing palettes. Modeling healthy choices is as important as the food served. This book delves into the dynamics of how your own eating habits can set the stage for your child's nutritional journey.

But our approach to food is not just about what's on the plate. Physical activity is an inseparable ally of nutrition, and we'll explore how this dynamic duo can work together for the benefit of your little ones. Furthermore, sustainability is not just a trendy buzzword—it's a core value that informs the way we should think about our food, from farm to fork.

Allergies and intolerances? Food labels? We're covering the challenges that come with dietary restrictions, as well as the strategies for ensuring your child's safety without compromising on nutritional quality or their sense of inclusion. And yes, that includes navigating social settings such as school cafeterias, birthday parties, and sleepovers!

We're also well aware of the snack conundrum—the daily tug-of-war between processed temptations and nourishing options. You'll discover an arsenal of creative ideas to make healthy snacking an enjoyable and routine part of your child's life.

Hydration plays a vital role in health, and it deserves as much attention as food. We'll delve into the importance of water, the impact of sugary drinks, and effective ways to make hydration a natural part of your child's day.

Culture adds another layer to the diverse tapestry of nutrition. This book advocates respect for diverse dietary traditions while balancing them with nutritional needs. Exploring the kitchen as a learning tool, we look to instill both culinary skills and nutritional knowledge through engaging cooking activities.

And in this digital age, technology is a potent ally. From apps to virtual communities, digital resources can support your efforts to educate and encourage healthy eating practices in interactive, enjoyable ways.

So, let's put on our aprons, roll up our sleeves, and prepare to construct the blueprint of a life enriched with flavorful nutrition and vibrant health for our children. There's no time like the present to make a positive impact that will last a lifetime.

Here's to happy, healthy eating adventures and the rich rewards that come from nurturing well-nourished children. Let's get started!

Chapter 1:
Foundations of Nutrition for Growing Bodies

As we delve into the world of childhood nutrition, let's lay the groundwork with a solid understanding of what makes up the building blocks of a child's diet. Just like constructing a sturdy house begins with a strong foundation, the health of our young ones starts with the essential elements of nutrition. In this chapter, we're tearing down complex scientific concepts and reconstructing them into digestible insights. We'll explore how the big three macronutrients—carbs, proteins, and fats—not only fuel those non-stop days of play but also act as the raw materials for growth and development. We won't forget the heavy lifters, the vitamins and minerals, which, despite being needed in smaller doses, are critical to keeping everything running smoothly, like spark plugs in an engine. And remember, this isn't a dry science lecture—it's the quintessential guide to nurturing future generations with every bite they take. So let's begin this refreshing journey into the foundations of nutrition—after all, it's the strongest roots that support the healthiest growth.

The Role of Macronutrients in the dialogue about children's nutrition is as essential and foundational as the blocks they use to build their playtime castles. Just like those interlocking pieces, macronutrients provide the fundamental support for growing bodies, anchoring a child's development and ensuring their health remains robust. But what exactly are these macronutrients, and why do they deserve our attention?

When we're talking about feeding our young ones, envision macronutrients as the trusty trio - carbohydrates, proteins, and fats. Each member of this nutrient band plays a crucial part in the symphony of growth, energy, and overall well-being. It's a performance we can't afford to ignore, especially when it comes to children.

Let's start with carbs, often painted as the villain in trendy diet books, but in reality, they're the main energy source for both kids and adults. It's about choosing the right kind - the complex carbohydrates found in whole grains, fruits, and veggies - which release energy steadily, keeping kids on the go without the dramatic highs and lows that come from sugary snacks.

Proteins step up as the body's building blocks, vital for the growth of muscles, organs, and even the enzymes that perform countless metabolic dances inside our bodies. For children, the right amount and quality of proteins are non-negotiable to ensure they are not only growing but flourishing.

Then there's fat, a macronutrient often misunderstood and unfairly rejected. Healthy fats - yes, there is such a thing - are key to developing brains and bodies. They help with the absorption of vital vitamins and provide a concentrated source of energy – essential for the unstoppable energy demands of a growing child.

One might ask, "How do these macronutrients come together in a child's diet?" It's a balancing act. Like any skilled juggler, we aim to keep all balls in the air – ensuring that children get the right mix of these essential nutrients. For a parent or caregiver, knowing this mix is as important as knowing the ABCs.

Children's bodies are like little factories that are always "on." They need a constant supply of energy to run, play, and learn. That's where carbohydrates come in strong, providing the fuel that keeps these factories humming. The objective here is to carefully pick carbs that provide not just energy but sustained nutrition - think whole grains like oats, brown rice, and whole wheat bread.

Imagine proteins as the foremen of the body's construction site. As children reach for the sky in their growth spurts, proteins ensure that their physical structure grows strong and stable. From lean meats and dairy to plant-based stars like beans and lentils, proteins must be a steady feature in the diet, and they're not just for muscle; they're also essential for brain development.

In our tales of nutrition, fats have been cast as the villain too often, but it's about time they were recognized for their heroics. While it's wise to keep a watchful eye on the amount and type of fat consumed, good fats like those found in avocados, nuts, and olive oil play a vital role in supporting cell growth and protecting vital organs. Plus, they make food taste great, which is always a bonus when you're coaxing a picky eater.

For busy parents, understanding the significance of macronutrients can be as simple as planning a well-rounded meal. It doesn't need to be a daunting daily chore. Small, deliberate choices can make a huge difference. Swapping out that white bread for a whole-grain alternative or choosing a handful of almonds over a bag of chips can steer those little bodies towards better health.

Moreover, the distribution of macronutrients throughout the day is crucial. Ever notice how a balanced breakfast can set the tone for a child's mood and energy level? It's like setting the right pace in a long-distance race – you want to keep the momentum without burning out. A breakfast rich in complex carbs and proteins with a smidge of healthy fats can do just that.

It's essential to remember that every child is unique, and so too are their nutritional needs. There is no one-size-fits-all approach here.

Some kids may have higher energy requirements because of their involvement in sports or other physical activities. Others may need different macronutrient ratios to support their metabolic rates. It's about observation, adaptation, and sometimes a little trial and error to find what works best.

When it comes to adolescents, the macronutrient plot thickens. Teenagers, with their rapid growth and often intense physical activity, require more of everything. It's like their metabolic engines shift into high gear, and they need quality fuel to match that intensity. It's not the time for empty calories; it's the time for nutrient-dense foods that provide the macronutrients they desperately need.

Educating kids early on about the value of macronutrients in their diet fosters a sense of nutritional autonomy and wisdom. We want to usher them towards making informed choices themselves, because one day, before you know it, they'll be the ones picking items off the grocery shelves or choosing their lunches at school.

Witnessing kids becoming more conscious of what fuels them is like watching a flower bloom - it's pure joy. A child who understands why a balanced plate matters is better equipped to face a world teeming with fast food and sugary temptations. They learn that what goes into their bodies affects not only how they feel today but how they grow and thrive in the years to come.

Lastly, let's acknowledge that we're living examples for the young eyes that watch us. When they see us enjoying a colorful salad or snacking on fruit and nuts, they're likely to follow suit. Our relationship with food mirrors onto them. Show them that eating well can be enjoyable and delicious, not a chore or a bore.

In sum, the role of macronutrients in a child's diet cannot be overstated. Like a well-rehearsed orchestra, each nutrient has its part to play, and the harmony they create together is what leads to a healthy, thriving child. Let's strive to make every meal a chance to teach our kids about the beauty and strength found in eating whole, nutritious foods. They're counting on us to pave the way for a lifetime of healthy choices - let's ensure we lead by example and with endless enthusiasm.

Carbohydrates, Proteins, and Fats for Kids - these three nutrients create the triumvirate of a balanced diet, heavily influencing the growth and development of our kids. In the fascinating world of nutrition, understanding how these macronutrients work in the bodies of our little ones is not only essential, it's empowering. So, let's peel back the layers and really dive into what carbohydrates, proteins, and fats mean for children's health.

First off, carbohydrates - these are not the enemy some paint them to be. In the lives of active, sprightly kids, carbs are the fuel that keeps engines running. Whole grains, fruits, and vegetables provide complex carbs that release energy slowly, ensuring a steadier blood sugar level and keeping those young minds alert and bodies lively throughout their action-packed days.

But here's the catch, not all carbs are created equal. While whole fruits offer fiber and essential nutrients along with their natural sugars, processed snacks bombard tiny bodies with a fast rush of energy that nosedives just as quickly. It's all about balance and choosing the right kind of fuel. Encouraging kids to snack on an apple instead of a candy bar can make all the difference in their focus, mood, and overall health.

Then, there are proteins, the building blocks of life. Proteins play a starring role in growth, repairing tissues, and helping the immune system to fight off invaders. A child's plate is incomplete without a source of lean protein, be it from animal or plant-based sources. Think grilled chicken, tofu, legumes, or even a handful of nuts (allergies permitting). Variety here is not just the spice of life, it also ensures a full spectrum of essential amino acids.

Parents, remember that kids have smaller stomachs. They need foods high in protein that aren't too bulky. A piece of fish might be better suited than a thick steak. Dairy products like milk, cheese, and yogurt are often a hit with kids and are another great source of protein, just keep an eye on the fat content.

Which brings us to fats. Ah, the much-maligned fat - it's not the villain many think it is. In fact, fats are absolutely vital for kids, particularly in supporting brain development and providing energy. But let's clarify something important - we're talking about healthy fats. The ones found in avocados, nuts, seeds, and fish like salmon are the gold standard. These unsaturated fats can promote heart health and support overall development without the negative impacts of their saturated comrades found in fried foods and many baked goods.

It's also worth highlighting that fat shouldn't dominate the plate but should complement the carbohydrates and proteins that are also present. You can sneak in healthy fats with a drizzle of olive oil on salad or by adding chia seeds to your child's morning oatmeal. Little changes like these can have big impacts on their nutrient intake.

Keep in mind, teaching kids about the balance of these macronutrients is as crucial as serving them. Explain in simple terms that like a car needs the right kind of gas to run, their bodies need the right kind of food to grow. It's about quality, quantity, and the perfect mix to keep our mighty little ones zooming around.

Furthermore, it's important to be mindful of each child's unique needs. Some kids burn through calories like wildfire, requiring more carbs and fats in their diet, while others may thrive with higher protein intake. It's about tailoring the menu to the child, keeping it as varied and colorful as their personalities.

Another dimension to consider is how these nutrients affect mood and energy levels. Ever dealt with a hyperactive child after a sugar rush?

Balance and choice in carbs, proteins, and fats can help stabilize energy levels, potentially leading to calmer, happier children with a steady supply of energy.

So, as you navigate this landscape with your kids, remember, it's not about excluding certain food groups or macronutrients; it's about understanding how to combine them effectively. A scoop of whole-grain rice, a palm-sized serving of grilled chicken, and a rainbow of veggies cooked with a spoonful of olive oil could be the ticket to a nutrient-packed, child-friendly meal.

Education is also key. Introduce your kids to the food groups as part of a game or an educational activity. Let them know that a superhero needs their strength (protein), their quick thinking (fats), and their energy (carbohydrates). Once they understand the superpowers each macronutrient brings to the table, they'll be more inclined to make healthier choices themselves.

Lastly, don't forget – moderation is key. It's okay for kids to have treats every so often. What's important is that they learn these are "sometimes" foods and not the foundation of their diet. This approach not only fosters a healthy relationship with food but can also instil a strong foundation for nutritional choices that can last a lifetime.

Hopefully, this exploration into carbohydrates, proteins, and fats for kids has painted a clear picture of the pivotal roles these macronutrients play. As guardians of our children's health, let's champion the cause, educate with joy, and lead by example. Here's to happy, balanced plates and even happier, healthier kids!

The Importance of Vitamins and Minerals As we delve further into the foundations of nutrition for growing bodies, we cannot overlook the vital roles that vitamins and minerals play. Understanding the significance of these nutrients is akin to unlocking a treasure chest for a child's well-being and development. It's not just about getting them to eat their greens – it's about nurturing their bodies and minds.

Vitamins and minerals are often referred to as micronutrients because the body needs them in smaller amounts compared to macronutrients like carbohydrates, proteins, and fats. However, don't let the term 'micro' fool you; these substances pack a mighty punch when it comes to a child's health. They are essential for robust immune systems, healthy brain development, and a plethora of bodily functions that contribute to a vibrant, energetic childhood.

Let's begin with vitamins – these organic compounds are crucial for normal growth and nutrition and are required in the diet because the body either doesn't produce them at all or not in sufficient quantities. Each vitamin plays a unique role; for instance, vitamin D works like a key, unlocking calcium's power to build strong bones and teeth, a critical element as children grow. The energizing B vitamins are instrumental for creating energy from the foods we eat and supporting the nervous system.

Now, onto minerals – these inorganic elements sourced from soil and water are just as vital. Calcium and phosphorus are the architects of strong bones, while iron is the very foundation of our blood, creating the hemoglobin that carries oxygen to busy, playing cells. Zinc is the shrewd guardian, bolstering the immune system and even helping wounds heal, so your little adventurer can get back to the business of exploring.

Envision the body as a complex machine – vitamins and minerals are like the nuts, bolts, and oil that keep it running at peak efficiency. Without them, processes start to falter, which can lead to deficiencies with very real impacts on a child's health. Iron deficiency, for instance, can result in anemia, a condition that brings on fatigue and affects concentration – hampering a child's ability to learn and play.

For those caring for children, it's vital to ensure their diets are rich in these micronutrients. Fortunately, nature offers a brilliant palette of foods – fruits, vegetables, nuts, seeds, whole grains, lean meats, and dairy products – that are brimming with vitamins and minerals. It's about creating a colorful plate, not just for aesthetics, but for a spectrum of nutrients to fuel growth and learning.

A common pitfall, however, is the reliance on vitamin and mineral supplements as a safety net for a poor diet. While they can be beneficial in specific cases, especially where individual deficiencies are identified, they can't mimic the complex, synergistic effects of whole foods. A chewable vitamin C tablet doesn't bring with it the fiber, flavonoids, and other compounds that an orange has, which together contribute to overall health.

Many parents and caregivers wonder how they can ensure their children are getting enough of these crucial nutrients. Start with regular meals and snacks that include a variety of food groups. Each group provides different vitamins and minerals; for example, leafy greens are excellent for vitamin K, while dairy products are a prime source of calcium. The answer lies in diversity – the more varied the diet, the more likely a child's nutritional needs will be met.

But what if your child turns up their nose at anything green or refuses to touch meat? This is where creativity in the kitchen comes into play. Blending spinach into a fruit smoothie or adding pureed vegetables into sauces and stews are clever ways to bolster nutrient intake without a battle of wills. Food presentation can also pique a child's interest – who wouldn't be curious about broccoli trees standing in a mound of mashed potato?

Learning and involving your child in food choices is another educational approach. Exploring farmers' markets, cooking together, and discussing where food comes from can demystify vegetables and fruits, making them more appealing. When children understand that carrots can help them see better at night, or that milk might help them grow strong like their favorite athlete, they're more likely to develop an interest in eating them.

It's also important to keep a watchful eye on your child's growth and development, as it can give clues to possible nutrient deficiencies. If a child seems lethargic, has dry skin, poor dental health, or frequent infections, it might be time to scrutinize their diet more closely or consult a healthcare professional to see if they're missing out on essential micronutrients.

Amid the whirlwind of raising kids, it's easy for vitamin and mineral intake to slip between the cracks, especially with picky eaters or those with food allergies or intolerances. Yet, with a little vigilance and a lot of variety, we can ensure these tiny dietary powerhouses do their job in growing healthy, happy kids.

As we journey through the different facets of a child's dietary needs, it's clear that vitamins and minerals are foundational elements. They might not get as much press as proteins or carbs, but they're the silent champions of growth and wellness. It's not just about feeding children; it's about nourishing them, one vitamin and one mineral at a time.

A Deep Dive into Micronutrients Having explored the macronutrients that form the bulk of our diet, let's zoom in on the often-overlooked but equally essential micronutrients. These are the vitamins and minerals that our bodies require in smaller quantities, yet they punch far above their weight in terms of their impact on a child's growth and development. When we talk about micronutrients, we're referring to a multitude of characters each playing a critical role in the complex dance of nutrition.

First off, let's get a handle on vitamins. These organic compounds are crucial for countless bodily functions, from supporting the immune system to ensuring proper vision. Picture vitamin A: it's not just about carrots improving your night sight, it's about a nutrient that supports cell growth and differentiation, particularly vital for growing bodies. Or the B vitamins, which are like a skilled symphony, each member conducting an aspect of energy production and allowing the body to utilize the energy from the foods we eat.

Then there's vitamin C, often touted for its role in immunity, but that's just the beginning. This vitamin is also a key player in collagen formation, helping heal those skinned knees from playground adventures. And let's not forget vitamin D, which we often associate with sunlight. Vitamin D assists in the absorption of calcium and promotes bone health, an absolute must for kids' lively activities and their growing skeletal framework.

Minerals are next on the roster. These inorganic elements come from soil and water and are absorbed by plants or consumed by animals. We've got the heavy hitters like calcium and phosphorus, which are the building blocks of strong bones. Then there's iron, which is like the cargo train of the bloodstream, transporting oxygen to every corner of the body. A well-oiled machine, our body needs iron in just right amounts to ensure our kids have the energy and focus whether they're in the classroom or on the soccer field.

Zinc is another star, playing a key role in growth, immune function, and wound healing. It's a multitasker that can't be ignored, especially as children encounter new germs and grow faster than we can keep up with. There's also the less-discussed but no less important selenium, a mineral that supports various bodily processes, including cognition, which is paramount when fostering the bright minds of future generations.

While maintaining an awareness of these micronutrients is vital, the next challenge is ensuring kids get enough of them through their diet. It's not always as simple as it sounds. Kids can be notoriously picky, and let's face it, a plate of kale doesn't always win the popularity contest. But it's not just about leafy greens; a colorful array of fruits and vegetables can help ensure a broad spectrum of micronutrients. Think of it as painting a rainbow on the plate, a culinary masterpiece rich in an array of vitamins and minerals.

It's also imperative to recognize that while deficiency in these nutrients can have significant consequences, so can an excess. The key is balance and variety. A diet that's too heavy in fortified foods or supplements might introduce more of a certain vitamin or mineral than necessary, which can, in some instances, be just as detrimental as a deficiency. This is where the idea of whole foods comes into play—nature's own packaging often provides these nutrients in just the right amounts.

As gatekeepers of our children's diets, we face the puzzle of ensuring these tiny nutrients don't slip through the cracks. Education is one of our best tools. Knowing that iron can be found in not only red meat but also in beans and lentils, or that bell peppers can offer even more vitamin C than oranges, empowers us to make informed food choices.

Supplementation might sometimes be necessary, especially when dealing with restrictive diets or specific health conditions. However, reaching for a supplement should be a considered choice, often best made in consultation with a healthcare provider to ensure it's in the best interest of the child's unique nutritional needs.

How do we navigate food preferences to ensure these important vitamins and minerals are consumed? Creativity is key. Smoothies can be an excellent way to incorporate a variety of fruits (and even some veggies) for a vitamin-packed punch. Sneaky chef tactics, like blending vegetables into sauces, can also help boost nutrient intake without a fight. And let's not forget the power of presentation – arranging foods in a fun, appealing way can entice kids to give them a try.

But above all, it's about instilling a sense of food exploration and appreciation in our little ones. When they understand the role of food as fuel and the concept of 'eating the rainbow' for health, they're more likely to adopt and maintain these habits as they grow. Sharing the 'why' behind the food choices can lead to a deeper understanding and cooperation.

Acknowledging the pivotal role of micronutrients in a child's diet doesn't require a degree in nutrition. It calls for a dash of curiosity, a sprinkle of diligence, and a hefty helping of patience. It's about diversifying the palate with a range of whole foods, each packed with their own unique set of micronutrients.

Finally, remember that nutrition is ever-evolving, and what we understand about it today may shift as we uncover more about the complex interplay of nutrients in our bodies. Keep abreast of new developments, but ground yourself in the time-tested wisdom that a varied, balanced diet rich in whole foods tends to be the golden ticket for getting those all-important micronutrients into our children's diets.

Arming our kids with a diverse and nutrient-rich diet is one of the greatest gifts we can offer. And while the landscape of child nutrition is vast and varied, with every small bite and every playful meal, we're setting the foundation for lifelong health and happiness. It's an investment that pays dividends in vibrant growth, boundless energy, and the joy of a vibrant life lived to the fullest.

Chapter 2:
Establishing Healthy Eating Habits Early On

After laying the essential nutritional groundwork, it's time to turn those foundations into sustainable actions. Knowing how vital the early years are to a child's development, establishing healthy eating habits from the start can set the scene for a lifetime of positive food choices. It's about creating a home where fresh, colorful, and whole foods are the norm, and where the occasional treat doesn't derail an otherwise balanced diet. With your guidance, children can learn to appreciate the taste and benefits of nutritious meals, making the wise choice the easy choice. Starting these habits early is key because as kids grow, they'll carry these behaviors with them, like hidden treasures in their health arsenal. The focus of this chapter isn't just about picking the right foods—it's about crafting an environment where healthy decisions flourish effortlessly, setting a routine that feels more like a rhythm than a rigid schedule. This chapter is your roadmap to ease your kids into a world where eating well is as natural to them as laughing and playing. So, let's nurture their well-being with joy and, rest assured, this investment will yield dividends for their future health.

Creating a Positive Food Environment As we journey together through the critical path of nurturing healthy eating habits in children, it is clear that the ambiance in which food is consumed is as pivotal as the food itself. In this space, not only do children eat, but they also form associations and develop attitudes toward food that last a lifetime. Crafting a positive food environment caters to the sensory experience of eating and can make the difference between a child reluctantly poking at their broccoli and one who dives in with enthusiasm.

At its core, a positive food environment is where nourishment and pleasure intersect. Here, children should feel encouraged to explore new textures and flavors without the pressure of a 'clean plate club' mentality. It's a space where healthy foods are easily accessible, and meal times are viewed as opportunities for connection rather than contention. This convivial setting encourages kids to be curious and develop preferences based on genuine enjoyment, not coercion or bribery.

Firstly, let's talk visibility and accessibility. Healthy options must be the easiest choices in the kitchen. Placing a bowl of fresh fruit on the counter and stocking lower pantry shelves with wholesome snacks encourages autonomy in kids' food selections. The principle is simple: what's in sight is in mind, which in turn finds its way onto the plate. This doesn't mean banishing treats outright, but rather promoting balance where more nutritious foods take center stage.

Collaboration during meal planning can also foster a sense of agency in children. Sitting down together to plan weekly meals instills a sense of involvement that can translate into excitement about eating. When children contribute to the decision-making process, they are more likely to invest in trying and enjoying the meals they helped create. This partnership makes dietary guidance mutual rather than prescriptive.

Dining together as a family cannot be undervalued in creating a positive food environment. Shared meals are platforms for role modeling balanced eating and for discussing the day's highlights and challenges. The focus is on the shared experience and not just the food, reducing the stress for children who may be less adventurous eaters.

Furthermore, family mealtime should be device-free to prevent distractions that can lead to mindless eating.

Speaking of adventures, theme nights can be an exciting avenue to introduce children to a variety of cuisines and nutrients. "Taco Tuesdays" or "Farmers Market Fridays" are not just fun, but also educational. Such events demonstrate the diversity of nutritious foods and can inspire a lifetime of curiosity about different cultures and flavors. Plus, they're a perfect moment to subtly incorporate those vegetables into a favorite dish.

Consistency is key, yet flexibility shouldn't be completely forsaken. Maintaining a structured schedule for meals and snack times provides the framework within which kids can predict and understand their eating patterns. Flexibility comes into play by allowing for occasional deviations like meals out or special treats, which help children learn moderation and the concept of occasional indulgences within a generally healthy diet.

Emphasizing variety, another cornerstone of a positive food environment, brings in a spectrum of vitamins and minerals essential for growth. A colorful plate is more than just visually engaging—it's a representation of a range of nutrients that benefit a child's body. Encourage kids to create a rainbow on their plate, and they'll likely remember the experience along with the health benefits.

Positive reinforcement also plays a role. Focusing on the positives of food choices ("You chose the carrots—great job getting your vitamin A for super vision!") rather than the negatives encourages children to repeatedly make healthful choices. This carrot, versus stick, approach lays the groundwork for a lifelong positive relationship with food.

Comfort in the environment also matters. Children should have a designated eating area that is comfortable and proportionate to their size. A child's dining space should allow their feet to touch the ground and the table to be at an appropriate height. Such tailored accommodations can make the eating experience more enjoyable and focused.

Education is an instrumental component of creating a healthy eating stage for kids. When they understand why their bodies need a variety of foods, they are more likely to make nutritious choices without perceiving them as a chore. Interactive learning opportunities, where children can touch, smell, and even help grow foods, will deepen their connection to what they eat.

Limiting negative food talk is crucial. Words can unintentionally cast a shadow over certain foods ("junk" food), creating a taboo allure that can lead to unhealthy binges. Instead, cultivate a language around food that is neutral and focuses on frequency ("sometimes foods") and balance rather than demonizing any particular item.

Mindfulness is another ingredient to sprinkle into your positive food environment. Teaching children to be mindful of their hunger cues, to savor their food, and to be present during meal times can prevent overeating and foster a healthy relationship with food. This mindfulness is not only about slowing down to chew; it's about appreciating the flavors, textures, and joy that food brings.

Lastly, navigating dietary preferences and allergies with sensitivity ensures that everyone feels included in the meal experience. Alternatives should not be considered an inconvenience but an opportunity to expand the collective palate of the family. Conscious inclusion sets the tone for empathy and understanding around food that kids will mirror in their own lives.

Remember, while it's important to nudge children towards nutritious choices, the goal is not to create a perfect eater, but to foster a positive association with a wide range of foods and eating experiences. Perfectionism can inadvertently cause stress and anxiety around meal times, defeating the purpose of a positive environment.

A positive food environment can make the world of difference in a child's development, setting the stage for a lifelong commitment to nourishing their body respectfully and joyfully. When the environment is right, healthy eating follows naturally, creating a pleasant rhythm that children will dance to well into their futures.

The Power of Routine and Consistency As we've seen, creating a positive food environment is a robust start toward nurturing healthy eating habits in children. Yet, the linchpin for truly ingraining these habits lies within an often overlooked but remarkably powerful approach: the establishment of routine and consistency. It's one thing to introduce wholesome foods to a child's diet; it's another to make them the cornerstone of daily consumption.

The comfort and predictability of a routine can't be overstated, especially when it comes to children. When we talk about establishing routines around meals, we're not suggesting a rigid schedule that can never be deviated from. Instead, think of it as a rhythmic pattern that children come to know and expect—a reliable cadence to the day that includes regular meal and snack times.

Consistency is the key to unlocking the benefits of a routine. It's about making healthy eating an expected part of every day, rather than a sporadic event. This constant repetition allows eating well to become second nature for children. Over time, they begin to associate meal times with not only hunger cues but also with a chance to nourish their bodies.

Routines help to establish clear guidelines for children and can significantly reduce mealtime battles. When kids are accustomed to eating breakfast, lunch, and dinner at similar times each day, their bodies adapt to this schedule. Their internal hunger signals sync up with the routine, promoting better appetite regulation which is an essential aspect of developing a healthy relationship with food.

With consistency comes a sense of security. The reliability of a routine gives children a sense of control and comfort. They know what to expect, and in the unpredictable world of a child, that can be a soothing anchor. It's important to maintain regularity not only in the timing of meals but also in what's offered. Having a variety of vegetables, fruits, whole grains, and lean proteins consistently served ensures these food groups become familiar and eventually preferred.

Of course, life isn't perfect. There will be days when routines are disrupted—special occasions, holidays, or simply life's unforeseen events. The beauty of a well-established routine is its resiliency. When children are grounded in regular healthy eating habits, these exceptions won't derail their nutrition journey, for they will naturally gravitate back to the familiar structure once the irregularity passes.

Implementing a consistent eating routine doesn't mean meals have to be monotonous or lack creativity. On the contrary, it can create a stable framework within which you can explore food diversity. Regularly introducing new foods within the established meal construct encourages children to be open-minded and adaptable eaters without overwhelming them.

How does one start building these routines? Simple: begin small. The addition of one consistent, healthy addition to each meal can make a difference over time. For instance, make it a habit to serve a vegetable with every dinner. The predictability of expecting a vegetable to appear on their plate each evening reinforces the norm that veggies are an integral part of dining.

Snack times are an excellent opportunity to reinforce the consistency principle. Instead of random snacking, scheduled snack times can regulate a child's hunger and avoid overindulgence. Offering the same array of healthy options during these times can familiarize young taste buds with nutritious choices.

The consistency in meal planning also extends to grocery shopping. When children see the same healthy items routinely being added to the shopping cart, it sets the tone for what constitutes everyday foods as opposed to the occasional treat. Involve children in this process, allowing them to pick from a selection of wholesome options; it will foster their investment in the routine.

Patience is a virtue when it comes to establishing any routine. It's common to encounter resistance initially, but perseverance pays off. Reinforce the routine with positive reinforcement, focusing on the wonderful flavors and how these foods make us feel—energized, strong, and happy. Pair this with an explanation of why these foods are beneficial, giving children a sense of empowerment over their choices.

One shouldn't underestimate the power of a shared family mealtime routine either. Families who eat together without the distractions of technology tend to have better dietary practices. This daily gathering is not just about eating—it's a ritual that nurtures both body and spirit, creating a communal experience that reinforces the value of nutrition.

Lastly, consistency must be reflected not just in when and what children eat, but also in how parents and caregivers model these behaviors. Children are incredibly perceptive and often mirror the eating patterns of the adults around them. If they see consistent, healthy eating behaviors in their role models, they are more likely to imitate them.

Routine and consistency are more than just methods for teaching children healthy eating habits. They are the steady drumbeat that sets the pace for a lifetime of nutritious living. As caregivers, when we embrace these principles, we're not just feeding children for a day; we're nourishing their future, one predictable, healthy bite at a time.

Chapter 3:
Planning Balanced Meals for Energetic Kids

As we pivot from establishing foundational eating habits, let's turn our attention to the nuts and bolts of meal planning—crafting balanced meals for our vibrantly energetic little ones. Kids are whirlwinds of activity, and their growing bodies need a symphony of nutrients to fuel their day-to-day adventures. It's all about mixing and matching food groups to create that color-filled plate that not only looks inviting but packs a nutritional punch. Think of it like painting a masterpiece, where each brushstroke represents a different nutrient group. We've got to balance our canvases with proteins that rebuild, carbs that recharge, fats that satiate, and vitamins and minerals that protect. And yes, we also sprinkle in some wizardry to weave those greens and beans into their meals without a standoff. It's not just about tossing together what's on hand—though there's an art to that too—but about intentional choices that support sustained energy, focus, and growth—all tailored to each kid's gusto for life. So let's roll up our sleeves and plan meals that are as dynamic and varied as the kids devouring them; meals that will have them dashing back for seconds before zooming off to their next grand escapade.

Designing the Mighty Kids' Plate When we talk about the Mighty Kids' Plate, what we envision is a vibrant canvas, a one-plate summary of balanced nutrition for our young ones. It's not just about piling on whatever is available in the fridge – it's an art form, combining colors, nutrients, flavors, and textures into something that not only feeds the body but also delights the senses and emboldens the spirit of our children.

In the world of childhood nutrition, there's a clear need for simplicity and structure. Kids are learning and exploring, so the plate in front of them should mirror that adventure. But how do you balance the ideal plate to support growth, provide energy, and promote lifelong healthy eating habits? This is where we roll up our sleeves and get to work.

To kick things off, let's reimagine the plate as a guide akin to a painter's palette. Half of this plate should spill over with a rainbow of fruits and vegetables. The allure here is two-fold: the visual appeal that piques curiosity, and the burst of vitamins, minerals, and fibers that come from fresh produce.

The other half of the plate? Well, that's where we bring in the support actors – grains and proteins. But not just any grains! We're talking whole grains that haven't been stripped of their nutritional value. Quinoa, brown rice, and whole wheat pasta are just a few star players. Then, we have proteins, but let's consider the variety – from animal proteins like fish and poultry to plant-based champions like beans and lentils.

Designing the plate with an eye for balance doesn't mean shunning fats either. Instead, we opt for the healthy kind, found in nuts, seeds, and avocados. These are essential but should be included with a thoughtful hand – a drizzle of olive oil on a salad, a smattering of nuts for added texture.

It's important to remember that kids are not miniature adults. Their energy needs are high and their bodies are growing. That's why on their plate, the food needs to be densely packed with nutrients, not just empty calories. It's about fueling those endless days of play, learning, and growth.

Now, while we're charting this culinary map, let's underscore the importance of dairy, or its alternatives, for a good dose of calcium and vitamin D. A glass of milk, a cube of cheese, or a dollop of yogurt can sail right next to the plate – essential for building strong bones and teeth.

Don't forget the power of herbs and spices either. They're like the secret code to getting kids hooked on flavors without the overload of salt and sugar. A sprinkle here and a dash there can transform a typical dish into a tantalizing experience that transcends mere nourishment.

When we break the plate down, the dimensions are equally crucial. Portion sizes should be realistic – we're not trying to see who can build the highest mountain of mashed potatoes. Tailoring portions to the child's age and activity level is vital, ensuring that they walk away from the table satisfied, not overstuffed.

Let's be real, though. You might have a plate designed worthy of accolades, but it's no good if the kids turn their noses up at it. Incorporating their preferences, involving them in meal planning, and making slight tweaks to introduce new foods can transform reluctance into excitement.

Variety is the spice of life, so let's keep that plate dynamic. Repeating the same foods can lead to boredom, so we should aim to rotate options regularly. Keep seasonal fruits and veggies in the mix and pair them with different grains and proteins to keep those taste buds guessing.

Remember, our aim isn't just to fill their bellies – it's to carve out a path to wise dietary choices. We want them to see their plate as an everyday adventure, an opportunity to discover new tastes, textures, and the joy of eating wholesomely.

Here's where we toss out the idea that healthy is synonymous with bland. Healthy can and should be mouthwateringly delicious. It's imperative that we as caregivers are mindful of the preparative processes – baking instead of frying, steaming instead of boiling to oblivion, and finding that delicate balance between nourishing and flavorful.

So let the Mighty Kids' Plate be a reflection of diversity – not just in the foods that make it up but in the cultural richness they can represent. Let your child's plate be a passport to the world, sampling whole foods from different cuisines, and adding yet another dimension to their growing palates.

Lastly, while fostering independence is crucial, guidance is key. We navigate this journey together with our children, holding their hands as they learn the ropes of healthy eating, gently nudging them along the path of nutritious and joy-filled dining experiences that set the foundation for a lifetime of well-being.

Let's embrace the construct of the Mighty Kids' Plate as an evolving tool, one that adapts and grows with our children, never rigid but always rooted in the principles of balance and good nutrition. It's through this lens we can shape not just meals, but habits and ideas around eating that nourish our kids today and far into their futures.

Portions and Food Group Ratios As we transition from addressing the macro and micronutrients essential in a child's diet, it's time to turn our attention to putting that knowledge into practice. Specifically, we're going to explore the portions and food group ratios that make up the meals served to our growing kids. This means delving into not just what we serve but how much of it ends up on those colorful little plates.

Understanding portion sizes is like having a superpower when it comes to feeding our kids. It allows us to ensure they're not overeating while still getting the nutrients they need from each food group. Let's paint a picture of this 'balanced plate.' Fruits and veggies should take up half the space. They're the stars of the show, bursting with vitamins, minerals, and fiber. Next is lean proteins; give these guys about a quarter of the plate – think poultry, fish, legumes, or tofu. They're key for muscle growth and repair.

Whole grains or starchy veggies should fill the remaining quarter. They provide that slow-releasing energy throughout the day—fuel for the fun. As for dairy or its alternatives, we're looking at including a portion comparable to a small cup, aiding in bone development with calcium and vitamin D. Now, keep in mind, the size of these portions isn't one-size-fits-all. They should scale with the child's age, activity level, and growth needs.

For a preschooler, a tablespoon per year of age can be a handy guide for serving sizes. It's simple and visual. As they grow into those busy school years, portions become more substantial, but the balance of the plate remains consistently varied. Let's not forget, though, kids' appetites can fluctuate, and forcing them to clear their plates can lead to overeating. Instead, let's encourage them to listen to their hunger and fullness cues, fostering a mindful relationship with food.

Now, food groups shouldn't live in isolation. A roasted sweet potato (hello, starchy veg!) becomes a flavor fiesta with a sprinkle of cinnamon and a dollop of Greek yogurt (protein and dairy ticked!). It's about creating a synergy of nutrients on the plate that also excites the taste buds.

One might ask, "What about fats?" These guys are important, too, for brain development and absorbing certain vitamins. But they're more like a garnish—think of drizzling olive oil over veggies or adding avocado slices to a wrap. They're present but not overwhelming the meal.

Speaking of ratios, while it's great to have this balanced plate model, flexibility is key. Some days the veggie intake might be lighter at lunch but can be compensated for at dinner. Same goes for protein or grains. It's the bigger dietary pattern that matters over the course of a week, not every single meal.

Moving on, let's nod to the fun stuff: treats. They're not front and center, but they don't have to be banished either. When sweets or less nutritious options make their way in, keeping portions small and infrequent helps maintain the overall harmony of the diet without swinging to extremes.

When it comes to family meals, sharing food can be an engaging way to understand portion control. Placing dishes in the center of the table and letting everyone serve themselves teaches kids to take what they need and recognize when they've had enough. It's also a chance for you to model good portion sizes for them to emulate.

Holidays and celebrations? These are times when the rules can relax a bit. It's perfectly okay for the food group ratios to shift during special occasions, making room for tradition and treats. It's what we do regularly that shapes children's habits, not the occasional divergence from the norm.

For those managing busy schedules, pre-plated or pre-portioned meals can be a godsend. They make it easy to maintain proper ratios without the hassle of measuring each time. Just tweak as needed for each child's appetite and development stage.

As kids grow, getting them involved in portioning out their meals can empower them. They learn the concept of balance and how to apply it practically. Pair this with swapping stories about everyone's day and you've got a recipe for successful mealtimes that are about nourishment and connection alike.

Lastly, while it's important to have these guidelines, it's just as important to keep the pressure low. Kids naturally have varying appetites and preferences, and that's okay. It's all about providing a variety of food groups at each meal, serving reasonable portions, and allowing kids the autonomy to hone their internal hunger and fullness meter.

The takeaway? Aim for a plate that represents the main food groups in satisfying, child-friendly portions. Keep it varied, keep it colorful, and above all, keep it fun. Watching these little ones flourish with the fuel you provide is rewarding beyond measure. It sets them on a path to making independent, healthy choices that will nourish their bodies and minds for years to come.

Armed with this understanding of portions and food group ratios, you're well on your way to crafting meals that are as balanced as they are delightful. So, take a moment to appreciate the joy of nutritionally savvy meal planning—it's an art and a science that garners a lifetime of benefits.

Snacking Smart for Sustained Energy - as we navigate the nuances of providing balanced meals for our dynamic youngsters, let's turn our focus towards a critical element of daily eating patterns: the snack. We must debunk the myth that snacking is inherently bad; it's not about snacking less, but about snacking smart. Kids have high energy needs and their smaller stomachs mean they may not always get enough fuel from meals alone. Smart snacking fills these gaps and maintains their energy levels.

Consider snacks as mini-meals that provide nutrients rather than just empty calories. Opt for whole foods, such as nuts, yogurt, fruits, and vegetables, which offer a wealth of nutrients alongside the calories they contain. The trick is to choose foods that are packed with fiber, protein, and healthy fats to promote satiety and sustain energy.

Understand the body's energy mechanism: Complex carbohydrates found in whole grains and legumes offer a steady release of energy, as opposed to the quick spike and crash that comes from more refined snacks. Pairing these with protein can help slow digestion and stabilize blood sugar levels, keeping those energy levels steady.

One can't ignore the implications of blood sugar levels in children's snacking habits. The highs and lows of sugar rushes are all too real and can have a tangible effect on their mood and concentration. Emphasizing the importance of low glycemic index snacks can help them maintain a stable and cheerful disposition throughout the day.

Timing of snacks matters as well. Offer snacks a few hours after a meal and at least an hour before the next one to prevent them from spoiling their appetite. This timing ensures they are truly hungry for their snacks and that each snacking opportunity is used to provide them with energy and nutrients they need to grow and learn.

Let's not overlook the power of hydration. Often, when kids think they are hungry, they might just be thirsty. Encouraging regular water intake will not only keep them hydrated but can also prevent overeating by helping to distinguish between hunger and thirst signals.

Don't let snacking be a passive activity. Encourage children to listen to their own hunger cues rather than eating out of boredom or because they see others eating. Mindful snacking helps them develop a healthy relationship with food and their own bodies' needs.

Make snacking fun and interactive. Involve the kids in preparing their snacks, maybe assembling a trail mix or topping a whole grain cracker with cheese and tomato. This engagement not only makes snacking more enjoyable but also serves as an educational experience in making healthy choices.

Consistency in snacking can also help manage energy levels. If children have a rough idea of when to expect a snack, it's easier for them to regulate their hunger and eating patterns through the day.

This doesn't mean snacks can't be spontaneous, but a routine can often prevent excessive hunger and overeating.

For the portable and hectic days, pre-packaged snacks can be a tempting option, but let's not fall into the convenience trap. With a little preparation, homemade or well-chosen wholesome snacks can be just as convenient and far healthier. Think whole fruit, homemade granola bars, or pre-sliced veggies in a to-go container.

Don't forget to rotate snack options regularly to avoid monotony. A colorful variety ensures a broader intake of nutrients and keeps children curious and engaged with their diet. This also paves the way for introducing new, perhaps even unexpected, healthy foods into their routine.

Snacks should complement, not compete with meals. By ensuring that they add to the nutritional quality of the day's food intake, rather than just filling up the gap with more of the same, you're setting the groundwork for a diverse, balanced diet.

Remember, the goal is not to have snacks replace meals but to maintain energy levels between them. It is about quality and timing, ensuring each snack has a purpose in the broader context of a day's nutrition. A well-crafted snack regimen is a powerful lever in a healthy lifestyle for growing kids.

In summary, smart snacking for sustained energy is a strategic endeavor. It calls for intentional choices, mindful timing, engaging variety, and an emphasis on nutritional value over mere calorie content. By instilling these principles in our children's daily routines, we nurture their growth and lifelong healthy eating habits.

As we close this section, let's carry forward the understanding that snacking is not the enemy of a balanced diet but, when done right, a faithful ally. It's these smart choices that can make all the difference, offering bursts of energy, nutrients, and joy in between life's daily adventures. Together, let's continue to support our mighty kids in making those smart snacking choices.

Chapter 4:
Overcoming Dietary Challenges

Weaving through the garden of nutrition for energetic kids, we stumble upon a prickly patch—dietary hurdles that seem to sprout overnight. It's quite the adventure to navigate a world where picky eaters reign and time ticks away faster than grains of quinoa in a salad spinner. Ah, but here we stand, equipped and ready to turn adversity into progress. As we've established robust food foundations from macronutrients to smart snacking, we're now stepping into the arena of *Overcoming Dietary Challenges*. This chapter isn't just about troubleshooting—it's where the rubber meets the road, empowering you with the resilience to meet your child's dietary needs head-on. Lively kids can be a tough crowd, presenting us with a kaleidoscope of preferences and schedules that are as packed as a lunchbox on a field trip. You see, it's not just about crafting the perfectly balanced plate; it's about making that plate fit into real, frantic life—dodging temper tantrums and tackling the tyranny of the clock. We'll explore tactics that resonate with the hustle of daily routines, transforming mealtime battles into victories crowned with broccoli florets. After all, raising a healthful eater is like cultivating a garden: it requires patience, persistence, and a whole lot of love. But fret not; as we roll up our sleeves and delve into this chapter, you'll gather strength from strategies designed for the busiest families, turning "I don't want that!" into "More, please!"

Coping with Fussy Eaters When it comes to dealing with fussy eaters, it's undeniable that patience is more than a virtue—it's a necessity. Parents and caregivers may at times feel like mealtime is a battleground, but with the right strategies, the table can turn into a place of exploration and, perhaps, even enjoyment. Let's delve into actionable ways to guide our choosy diners without turning dinnertime into a stressful event.

Start by understanding that fussiness is often a phase, a normal part of children's development as they exercise autonomy and express preferences. Rather than a source of frustration, this can be seen as an opportunity to instill healthy habits. It's also important to pinpoint specific dislikes and preferences. Is it a texture, a flavor, or a temperature issue? By getting to the root of the aversion, you can craft a nuanced approach to tackle it.

Never force a child to clean their plate. Coercion can create a power struggle and negative associations with eating. Instead, encourage them to try 'just one bite' with the understanding that it's okay if they don't like it. This one-bite rule eases the pressure and opens the door to new foods without demanding an immediate love for them.

Create a mealtime routine that involves set eating times. This helps regulate your child's hunger cues and sets the stage for more predictable eating behaviors. Fussy eaters often find comfort in knowing what to expect, and a routine can provide that security.

When introducing new foods, consistency is key. It may take several exposures to a new food before a child accepts it. Pairing the new food with familiar favorites can also ease the transition. During this process, stay neutral in your reactions; while enthusiasm can be encouraging, overly dramatic responses to rejection may inadvertently reinforce picky behavior.

Explore the power of choice. Giving your child a say in what's on their plate can make them feel empowered. Ask them to choose between two healthy options. This simple act of giving them control can improve their willingness to eat.

Get them involved in meal planning and cooking. When children take part in preparing their meals, they're more likely to be interested in eating them. It can be something simple like tearing lettuce for a salad or choosing the vegetables to include in a dish. Their personal investment can override their fussiness, at least to some extent.

Presentation matters. Fussy eaters might be more inclined to eat something that looks appealing or fun. Try to make the presentation of meals visually inviting for a child. For instance, arranging a face with vegetables on a plate or using cookie cutters for sandwich shapes can make healthy foods more enticing.

Sometimes, it's not about the food, but the environment. Eating together as a family, without distractions like TV or smartphones, can encourage better eating habits. It provides a relaxed atmosphere where the focus is on the meal and the pleasant company, which can sometimes coax a fussy eater to try something new.

Positive reinforcement can go a long way. Praise your child for trying a new food, no matter the result. This doesn't mean showering them with excessive accolades, but rather acknowledging their effort and bravery in tasting something outside their comfort zone. Avoid using food as a reward, as this can foster an unhealthy relationship with food.

Offer the same meals to everyone. Making a separate meal for the fussy eater implicitly suggests that it's okay to be picky. By serving one meal for the family, you normalize the eating experience and set a communal standard.

Vegetables and fruits can be particularly challenging for fussy eaters. Incorporate these vital food groups by blending them into smoothies or adding them into sauces where their presence is less pronounced. This covert approach can help meet nutritional needs while gently acclimating taste buds.

It's essential to stay calm and avoid power struggles during meals. The more attention is drawn to fussy eating behavior, the more likely it is to continue. Remember, this too shall pass. Most children outgrow their pickiness over time, especially with gentle encouragement and repeated exposures to a variety of foods.

For extremely fussy eaters, where weight loss or compromised growth is a concern, or eating issues seem to extend beyond typical picky eating, consulting a pediatrician or a nutritionist might be necessary. A professional can assess the situation and offer tailored advice or intervention if needed.

In summary, coping with fussy eaters is a mix of patience, creativity, and persistence. Remember, you're not alone on this journey. Countless parents and caregivers have navigated this territory, and with time, empathy, and some clever tactics, progress is not just possible—it's probable. Together, we can turn mealtime from a challenge into a stepping stone toward lifelong healthy eating habits.

Strategies for Busy Families For parents juggling careers, childcare, and the countless other demands of daily life, finding the time to plan and prepare healthy meals can often feel like an insurmountable task. Yet, even in the whirlwind of our packed schedules, it's vital we grasp the reality: The health of our children is paramount, and nutrition cannot be overlooked. Don't let busyness become a barrier to cultivating healthy eating habits in your little ones. Let's walk through a suite of strategies to keep your family's nutrition on track, even when time is at a premium.

Firstly, let's talk meal planning. It's not as daunting as it seems, and it doesn't necessarily mean slaving away in the kitchen for hours. Dedicate a small chunk of your weekend to sketch out the week's meals. Aim for variety, and include meals that can last more than one day. Think stews, casseroles, and hearty salads. If the idea of planning an entire week is overwhelming, start with three days at a time.

Batch cooking plays a role here as well. Cooking large quantities at once and storing portions for later use is a true game-changer for busy households. Double up on recipes and freeze the extras. This isn't just about main meals, either. Batching breakfast items like pancakes or muffin tin frittatas can save your mornings from chaos.

An often-missed shortcut is prepping ingredients in advance. A few moments spent chopping veggies, pre-cooking grains, or marinating proteins can significantly expedite meal prep during the weekday rush. Storage is key; invest in good-quality airtight containers that keep prepped food fresh.

In the heat of the week, simplicity is your ally. Adopting one-pan or one-pot recipes not only reduces the cook time but also the cleaning time. Dishes like stir-fries and sheet pan roasts are nutritious, quick, and involve minimal cleanup. Plus, you can tailor the ingredients to suit your family's taste buds and dietary needs.

The slow cooker is indeed a busy family's best friend. It's a set-and-forget approach to cooking, where you can throw in all the ingredients in the morning and come home to a delicious, ready-to-eat dinner. Kid-friendly favorites include slow cooker chili, tender pot roasts, and creamy chicken and rice.

Leftovers deserve more recognition. A slightly larger dinner can easily become the next day's packed lunch. With a little creativity, last night's roast chicken can heroically transform into a sumptuous chicken salad wrap or a savory rice bowl. Encourage your children's input; they might enjoy inventing new meal ideas.

For those days when cooking is out of the question, keep a stash of healthy staples that can be quickly assembled. Canned beans, pre-washed greens, and whole grain wraps can be lifesavers for pulling together a meal in minutes. Even rotisserie chickens from the supermarket can be part of a wholesome meal when combined with fresh veggies and brown rice or quinoa.

Involve the kids in meal preparation whenever possible. This can be an educational and bonding experience, plus it helps them develop an appreciation for what goes into their food. Younger children can wash produce or mix ingredients, while older ones can help chop and cook. It's an investment in fostering their life skills and interest in nutrition.

The power of the freezer cannot be overstated—stock it with frozen fruits and vegetables that can be easily added to dishes to increase their nutritional value. Blending a handful of spinach into a morning smoothie or stirring frozen peas into a pasta dish injects a boost of nutrients without any fuss.

Making a grocery list and sticking to it prevents impulsive purchases of less healthy options. Shopping with a plan also saves time and streamlines your store visits. If time constraints make shopping difficult, consider online grocery delivery services or curbside pickups that can fit into your busy life. Some families may also find community-supported agriculture (CSA) boxes a convenient and fresh option.

For snacks, pre-portion nuts, seeds, fruit, or whole-grain crackers for grab-and-go ease. Having these ready-to-eat snacks on hand staves off the temptation for you or your kids to reach for high-sugar, high-fat options when hunger strikes unexpectedly.

And let's not forget hydration. A water bottle for each family member encourages drinking water throughout the day, which is especially important for active kids. Feel free to infuse it with fruits or herbs to add a splash of flavor and entice them to sip more often.

Lastly, remain flexible. Some days will not go to plan, and that's alright. It's about creating a framework of healthy habits, not a rigid regime. If pizza night rolls around after a particularly hectic day, balance it out with a side salad and focus on a healthier day tomorrow.

Remember, every small step counts. Persistence and patience are key when finding your rhythm with meal planning and preparation. Soon enough, these strategies will settle into routine, benefiting not only the health of your children but also nurturing a happier, less stressed family environment.

Set a goal to implement one to two tips from this list each week. By steadily incorporating these strategies into your lifestyle, your family will inch closer to nutritional success, no matter how busy life gets. So, take a deep breath, gather your resources, and transform mealtimes from a hectic must-do into opportunities that nourish body, mind, and the family bond.

Chapter 5:
Parents' Influence on Children's Food Choices

As we peel back the layers of dietary behaviors, we find that parents are at the core of children's food preferences. You wield a spoon that's both a magic wand and a guiding rudder: with each meal, you're sculpting not just palates but lifelong habits. Picture this—it's not just the food on their plates that kids are gobbling up, but your attitude and choices as well. Each crunch and every munch is a lesson absorbed; your reach extends from the grocery aisles to the dinner table, casting a mold that sets rapidly and holds fast. While we'll dive into strategies like modeling healthy eating and tackling the dynamics at play within the family unit in subsequent sections, it's key to remember here that you're the chief taste-tester and trendsetter in your child's world of flavors. The art of balancing nutrition with nurturing, guidance without groans, is a subtle one, but the payoff is a bounty of lifelong healthy choices. So, let's take a heartfelt look at how your fork—and the path it carves—can foster a garden of nourishing habits for the tiny taste explorers in your life.

Modeling Healthy Eating As we pivot our focus toward the influential role parents and caregivers have on children's food choices, let's delve into the heart of this impact: modeling healthy eating. You've likely heard it said that children are like sponges, soaking up the world around them, and this couldn't be truer when it comes to dietary habits. When adults consistently choose nutritious foods and maintain a balanced diet, they set a silent, powerful example for the younger generation witnessing their choices daily.

Consider your everyday meal choices as a teaching opportunity. As you reach for a piece of fruit instead of a sugary treat for a snack, you're silently communicating the value of food selection based on nutrition. Don't underestimate the ripples of such actions; they can build into waves of healthy habits that carry your child into adulthood.

Many believe that discussing the importance of fruits and vegetables is enough, but actions resonate louder than words. If a child sees their guardian opting for a salad over fast food, they start to recognize healthy eating as a normal behavior. Let's not rely solely on school programs or occasional nutrition talks to get this message across when the dinner table can be one of the most impactful classrooms.

Indeed, reinforcements are foundational. A 'do as I say and as I do' approach lends credibility to your guidance on eating well. When you prioritize nutrition in your diet, you are showing—not just telling— kids that health is not an afterthought but a way of life. Parents can elevate this by involving kids in meal planning and explaining why certain foods make it onto the plate and others don't.

Have you noticed your child eyeing your plate? They're curious if what's good for them is also good for you. Share the same meals to validate that there's no 'kids food' and 'adult food,' only 'healthy food' that everyone enjoys. This sense of unity can be comforting and encouraging for children; they're part of the team, and everyone is working towards the same goal of wellness.

Acknowledge that no one's perfect, and balance does not mean perfection. An occasional indulgence showcases a healthy relationship with all foods—some are everyday foods, while others are treats. It's the proportions and frequency that matters. If you demonstrate balance, children grasp that they don't have to fear or avoid certain foods entirely; it's about context and overall patterns.

Let's highlight the importance of self-care through food. Discussing how a balanced meal benefits your body and mind can instigate open conversations about nutrition. Share how you feel after eating a hearty bowl of vegetable-rich stew versus a greasy meal. This kind of dialogue can develop into intrinsic motivation for children, as they start associating good food with feeling fantastic.

Body image and self-esteem are delicate subjects that often tie into discussions around eating; healthy modeling transcends diet and touches upon self-perception. Avoid vocalizing negative comments about your body or food guilt. Children quickly pick up on these sentiments and may start to mirror them. Display a positive attitude that celebrates all body types and focuses on eating for health, not just appearance.

Nutrition isn't solely about the food you eat, but also the atmosphere in which you dine. Create a pleasant environment free from distractions such as smartphones and televisions. Making mealtime a moment for engagement and interaction encourages thoughtful eating. It encourages kids to be mindful and attentive to how they fuel their bodies.

When the holidays arrive laden with special treats and traditions, use these occasions as a platform to teach moderation and the enjoyment of food without overindulgence. It's a fine balancing act to honor time-honored delights while also staying true to your everyday philosophy of health and nourishment.

Transparency around food choices, including discussing nutritional labels or why you buy certain items, provides kids with the knowledge to make informed decisions. It's one thing to fill the cart with vibrant, whole foods, but sharing the 'why' behind these selections reinforces the lessons you're living out.

What could possibly be even more convincing than simply modeling healthy eating? Making it fun! Explore new fruits and vegetables together, cook meals as a family, or engage in friendly taste tests. This lessens any pressure around new foods and lays a foundation of excitement and exploration around eating well.

However, remember to tune into your child's feedback. If they seem to resent or resist your guidance, it's crucial to step back and assess. Are you being too prescriptive? Is the message feeling less like inspiration and more like instruction? The journey towards healthy eating must be truly collaborative to be fruitful.

Even when dining out, pick restaurants that offer wholesome choices and reflect on the decisions being made. When children witness you navigating a menu with health in mind, the skill of making nutritious choices despite more indulgent options becomes less daunting for them.

And finally, consistency is key. Model healthy eating as a routine, not a phase. Children will carry these regular habits with them as they grow older. Your steadfast approach to nutrition demonstrates that healthy eating is attainable and sustainable, setting the stage for a lifetime of wellness.

In essence, be the mirror you wish your child to reflect. Your everyday choices paint a picture of health that children will instinctively want to echo. Consciously modeling healthy eating isn't just about what's consumed; it's about shaping a perspective that values nutrition, balance, and a positive relationship with food. It's about walking the talk, plate by plate, day by day.

Navigating Food-Related Family Dynamics As we peel back the layers of influence surrounding children's eating habits, we land squarely at the dinner table with a subject as tender as the vegetables we hope to serve: family dynamics. Within the family unit, an intricate web of attitudes, beliefs, and behaviors collectively shapes a child's relationship with food. This setting, where memories and meals are shared, becomes the foundational platform for lifelong eating patterns. Let's embark on a journey to traverse these intricate dynamics, unravelling strategies to steer the family ship towards the shores of healthy eating, without sparking a mutiny.

Eating together as a family can be a blissful symphony or resemble a cacophony of clashing cutlery, depending on the dynamics at play. One common scenario is the tug-of-war between a parent's nutritional aspirations for their child and that child's own food preferences. To navigate this dynamic, communication is key. Engage children in discussions about food, emphasizing the 'why' behind healthy choices. This open dialogue builds trust and understanding, rather than solely enforcing rules.

Another layer to navigate is varying food preferences across family members. It's a challenge akin to juggling apples and oranges, ensuring each person's dietary needs and likes are considered. Implementing taste tests or assigning 'theme days' can be a fun way to introduce variety and inclusiveness in meal planning. Encourage family members to contribute ideas, which fosters ownership and reduces pushback at mealtime.

Mealtime can also become a battleground when dealing with fussy eaters, demanding a strategic approach. Instead of framing it as a war over wills, approach it with empathy and patience. Offer a range of healthy options and let children have a say in what goes on their plates, within reason. Consistent exposure without pressure can eventually wear down resistance.

The intergenerational sharing of food traditions plays a substantial role in family dynamics. Grandparents, and parents, often pass down culinary customs that may not align with current nutritional guidelines. To respect tradition while prioritizing health, engage in gentle, respectful conversations about tweaking recipes or introducing new, healthier alternatives alongside the old favorites.

Family celebrations tend to revolve around rich, indulgent foods, which can set a precedent for associating festivities with overeating. Balance these occasions by also celebrating with active family outings or involving children in making healthier versions of traditional dishes. This teaches that enjoyment and food aren't exclusively interlinked with indulgence.

Each family member's dietary needs, whether due to age, health, or lifestyle, complicate the menu. Young athletes, for example, have different requirements than their sedentary siblings. Personalize portions and sides while maintaining a common core meal to simplify this complexity. This ensures everyone's needs are met without cooking separate meals for each person.

The role of caregivers and siblings can't be understated in influencing a child's eating behavior. Children often emulate older siblings and adults, so it's crucial for everyone to model positive eating habits. Treat this as an opportunity for collective betterment, where everyone's efforts, including children's attempts to make healthy choices, are recognized.

Let's not overlook the subtle, yet powerful force of emotional dynamics. Food is often used as a reward or consolation, creating an emotional attachment that can lead to overeating or comfort eating. Foster a neutral stance where food isn't a currency for affection or behavior but just one part of a larger healthy, active lifestyle.

Managing conflicting information from external sources like media, friends, or extended family members requires a united front. Establish clear, consistent messaging at home about your family's food values. Empower children with knowledge to make their own informed decisions when faced with external influences.

Setting boundaries can spur resistance, especially in teens seeking independence. Navigate this by involving them in decision-making processes, giving them some control over their dietary choices within the framework of healthy options. This respect for their burgeoning autonomy will help mitigate conflict and encourage responsibility.

Holiday meals and special occasions pose their own navigational challenges. Balancing tradition with health can be tricky, but it's an opportunity to instill moderation and mindfulness. By focusing on the social aspect of gathering and the joy of tasting various foods, children learn to appreciate food without overindulging.

Within blended or non-traditional family structures, aligning eating habits may seem like stitching a quilt from different fabric patches. Respect and patience are essential as new members bring in their unique food cultures and habits. Start new traditions that blend the old with the new, creating a cohesive, inclusive mealtime environment.

Lastly, handling resistance to change is like tending a garden; it requires nurturing and time. Rushing the process or forcing change can backfire. Make incremental changes and celebrate small victories to ensure the whole family gradually adopts a healthier lifestyle together.

To wrap up, successfully navigating food-related family dynamics means balancing respect for individual preferences with the aim of achieving collective health goals. It involves ongoing dialogue, flexible approaches, and a generous serving of patience. When the family unit functions harmoniously, it shapes a supportive environment where children can flourish and form positive lifelong eating habits.

In the end, remember, it's about progress, not perfection. Transforming family meals into nurturing experiences that support healthy choices is a journey worth taking, filled with opportunities to grow together. And as this tapestry of family dynamics continues to evolve, so will your approach to guiding children towards a lifetime of nutritious eating, one meal at a time.

Chapter 6:
The Significance of Physical Activity

As we turn the page from the foundations of nutrition, let's lace up our sneakers and step into the invigorating world of physical activity—a pillar just as crucial as diet for nurturing robust health in kids. It's common knowledge that kids brim with energy, and channeling this vigor through active play, sports, and family outings isn't just fun—it's essential for their physical and cognitive development. Think of exercise as the yin to nutrition's yang, a harmonious blend that forges resilient bones, sharpens minds, and cultivates habits that can hold up a lifetime of well-being. It's not just about the sweat and the number of steps on a pedometer. It's the laughter on the playground, the perseverance on the field, and the joy in moving that lifts their spirits and bolsters their hearts. In this chapter, we explore how integrating movement into daily routines can enrich the overall health landscape for our children, making the nutritious meals we serve them even more powerful. Together, nutrition and exercise weave the fabric of a lifestyle that can protect and propel our kids into a thriving future. They'll learn to love the way their bodies feel in motion, and that's a love that can carry them far.

Exercise and Nutrition: A Dynamic Duo As we've delved into the fundamentals of nutrition and the strategies for fostering healthy eating habits in kids, we've laid a robust foundation. But what about the role of physical activity? The coupling of exercise and nutrition underpins a child's overall health, development, and well-being. These two elements work synergistically, each amplifying the benefits of the other. They're the two wings that can help children soar to heights of optimal health and vitality.

Think of the body as a finely tuned engine. Nutrition provides the fuel, while exercise ensures that the engine runs smoothly and efficiently. When kids eat a balanced diet, they're armed with the essential energy and nutrients necessary to thrive physically. Exercise, then, is the ignition that turns potential energy into kinetic, realizing the power of those nutrients.

Engaging in regular physical activity from an early age establishes patterns that can last a lifetime. It strengthens muscles and bones, enhances coordination, and promotes healthy growth. Beyond the physical, exercise also offers powerful cognitive and emotional benefits. From increasing concentration and academic performance, to reducing symptoms of depression and anxiety, staying active is a core component of a healthy, happy childhood.

But how much exercise do kids need? Generally, it's recommended that children get at least an hour of moderate to vigorous physical activity every day. This includes a variety of activities that they enjoy and that get them moving in different ways – running, jumping, climbing, dancing, the list goes on. It's about finding that sweet spot where movement doesn't feel like a chore, but rather like an extension of play.

On the flip side, nutrition can significantly affect a child's energy levels and physical performance. A diet rich in whole foods such as fruits, vegetables, whole grains, lean proteins, and healthy fats furnishes the body with a spectrum of nutrients conducive to growth and energy production. Well-nourished kids have the stamina to be active and the building blocks to recover and grow stronger after physical exertion.

Moreover, studies have shown that when children combine regular physical activity with healthy eating, they are more likely to maintain a healthy body weight. Obesity in childhood is a growing concern, and it makes the partnership between movement and nutrition all the more crucial. By setting the standard for energy balance – the equilibrium between calories consumed and calories expended – we aid in the prevention of childhood obesity.

That being said, instilling these habits is not just about warding off weight issues. Exercise and nutrition are about nurturing every aspect of a child's health. Adequate hydration also plays a significant role here, complementing the duo of diet and physical activity. Keeping kids hydrated ensures that their bodies can perform optimally, especially during exercise or in warmer climates.

Parents and caregivers can foster this dynamic duo by being role models. When kids see adults in their lives valuing and enjoying physical activity – choosing to take the stairs instead of the elevator, going for family bike rides or hikes, participating in sports or dance – they're more likely to adopt these behaviors themselves. The same goes for healthy eating; witnessing adults making balanced meal choices encourages kids to follow suit.

It's also worth considering the timing and composition of meals in relation to activity. Offering a snack that includes a mix of carbohydrates and protein after exercise can help refuel and repair young bodies. For instance, giving a child a banana with a spoonful of peanut butter provides quick energy from the fruit and sustained energy from the fats and protein in the nut butter.

But the benefits aren't all long-term. In the immediate, kids who exercise regularly and eat well are usually more alert, have better moods, and can concentrate more effectively. These advantages translate into better performance at school and in extracurricular activities, as well as increased self-esteem and confidence.

There's potential for creativity in combining exercise and nutrition education, too. Take, for example, a garden project that incorporates physical work with lessons on plant-based nutrition. Kids are more likely to eat fruits and vegetables that they have a hand in growing, and the physical labor of gardening is great exercise. It's a win-win situation.

Perhaps most importantly, exercise and nutrition build upon each other to develop resilience. Kids who are physically active and well-nourished are better equipped to fend off illnesses, manage stress and recover from setbacks. They're prepared not only for the physical demands of life but the mental and emotional ones as well.

To wrap it up, if we envision a future where our children embody healthy lifestyles, we must recognize that exercise and nutrition are inseparable companions on this journey. They are the dynamic duo that, when harmonized, can spell the difference between a child just getting by and one who's thriving. So, let's encourage our kids to move their bodies, fuel them with the best nutrition possible, and watch them grow into healthy, well-rounded individuals.

In our next exciting chapter, we'll delve into the importance of incorporating movement into daily life, exploring various fun and effective ways to ensure our kids stay active in ways that fit seamlessly into the family routine. Let's keep the momentum going and foster a love for the active life in our kids!

Incorporating Movement into Daily Life Often, when we think about nurturing healthy habits in children, the focus tends to rest squarely on what they're eating. But let's shift gears and underscore another critical aspect of a healthy lifestyle—physical activity. Just as vital nutrients lay the building blocks for a strong body, regular movement fortifies these foundations and brings a plethora of benefits to the table, or in this case, the play park!

Understandably, the hustle and bustle of daily life can make weaving in regular physical activity seem like a tall order. However, with creativity and commitment, it's not only possible, but it can also be a joyous part of your routine. Let's explore ways to inject more movement into your kids' lives without it feeling like another daunting task on the checklist.

Firstly, consider the power of starting young. Kids are naturally energetic and curious, so take advantage of this by encouraging play that involves physical exertion. For toddlers, this could mean crawling through homemade obstacle courses. For older children, it might be climbing on jungle gyms or playing tag with friends. These sorts of activities help children develop motor skills and establish exercise as a fun and normal part of daily life.

Another key strategy is to lead by example. Children emulate the behavior of the adults around them. If they see you being active and enjoying it, chances are they'll want to join in the fun. Whether it's a weekend family hike, a quick game of basketball before dinner, or a dance-off in the living room, show them that exercise isn't just good for you—it can also be a blast.

Rethink transportation when possible. If safety and distance permit, encourage walking or biking to school instead of driving. The fresh air in the morning can wake up the mind just as well as it exercises the body. Even for short trips to the store or park, make locomotion part of the adventure. It's not just eco-friendly—it's body-friendly, too.

Don't overlook household chores—yes, really! While they may not be as exhilarating as other activities, tasks like sweeping, raking leaves, or washing the car involve body movements that count as physical activity. To make it more appealing, turn them into games or set up a reward system. An added bonus? Children learn responsibility and the value of contributing to the household.

Schedule 'active' playdates. While it's fine for kids to have some downtime with friends, suggest outings that involve movement. It could be anything from a visit to the trampoline park to a swimming session at the local pool. These social occasions then become opportunities for exercise, forming associations between fitness, fun, and friendship.

Let's not forget the importance of downtime and balanced routines. While embedding movement into daily life, remember to allow for rest. Children need unstructured time to relax and recharge. Leading an active lifestyle isn't about non-stop motion; it's about finding harmony between activity, play, and rest.

In the classroom setting, advocate for regular breaks where students can get up and move. This doesn't necessarily mean disrupting lessons; simple stretch breaks or a few minutes of 'brain gym' exercises can suffice to get the blood flowing and improve concentration.

When it comes to technology, there's a place for it in encouraging activity. Use pedometers or fitness trackers designed for kids to spark a bit of healthy competition. Many devices turn step counting into a game and can motivate kids to move more. Additionally, family-friendly fitness apps or active video games can provide guided workouts or dance routines for an indoor option.

Bond over active hobbies or sports. Find an activity that fits your child's interests and abilities and join them. Whether it's martial arts, soccer, or rock climbing, having shared interests can deepen your connection and ensure regular participation. Remember, the goal is to cultivate a love for movement that will last a lifetime.

If you're dealing with variations in weather, get creative indoors. Set up a mini circuit in your living room or have indoor 'olympics' with games that involve jumping, crawling, and balancing. You can also use household items like cushions for hopping over or yarn for makeshift limbo. When it rains outside, let the games begin inside!

For those children who are less inclined towards physical exertion, aim to incorporate incidental activity. This means finding ways to move that don't necessarily feel like exercise. It could be as simple as standing while doing homework, jumping rope during commercials, or taking the dog for a brisk walk.

Lastly, celebrate the wins, no matter how small. Hit 10,000 steps? Do a little victory dance. Climbed the jungle gym for the first time? High-fives all around. Positive reinforcement can work wonders in motivating children to stay active.

With this in mind, flip the script on 'exercise.' Instead of it being one more thing on the to-do list, view it as a treasured part of your day to connect with your kids and instill in them a vibrant, active lifestyle. It's about building a lifelong journey of health and well-being, step by playful step.

So, in wrapping up these tips, remember the aim is not to carve out extra hours in an already packed schedule but to integrate movement seamlessly into the routine. Model zest for life and physical vitality, and you'll likely find that your children will follow suit, reaping the benefits for years to come. As you can see, incorporating movement into daily life for kids isn't just about keeping them fit—it's about setting the stage for a balanced, vibrant, and joyful life.

In the next steps of our journey, we'll look at how a sustainable approach to eating not only benefits health but also our planet. As we foster these habits in children, we're nurturing responsible, informed individuals who care for themselves and the world around them.

Chapter 7:
Sustainable Eating Habits for the Planet and Our Children

In the rhythm of busy lives and the quest to feed our kids the best, we're now turning the page to a chapter that resonates with the heartbeat of our planet. Sustainable eating isn't just a trendy catchphrase; it's a profound commitment to the health of our Earth and the future of our little ones. Every meal we serve is a chance to nourish not only our children but also to respect the intricate ecological balance that sustains us. Let's peel back the layers of how our food choices impact the planet, revealing a tapestry woven with the threads of local produce, less meat, and waste-conscious consumption. Picture a world where our kids are not only culinary savvy but eco-warriors at the dining table—a world where each forkful is a statement of care for themselves and the environment. It's about embracing whole, plant-based foods that are as good for the land as they are for our bodies, minimizing our carbon footprint without sacrificing flavor or nutrition. So, let's seed the future with sustainable habits that blossom into a legacy of health for our children and generations to come.

Understanding the Impact of Food Choices As we transition from grasping the basics of nutrition for young individuals, it's paramount to recognize the ripple effect of our everyday decisions about food. It's not just about filling plates; it's about shaping lives, influencing health, and considering our environment. So, let's uncover the profound influence our food choices have on both personal health and broader ecological implications.

Dietary choices are more than just personal preferences; they're threads in a larger tapestry of health outcomes. For children especially, these choices set the groundwork for their growth and development. Nutrient-density is a term you'll hear often, and it's essential in assessing the value of foods consumed. Opting for kale over candy might seem an obvious choice, but it's not just about avoiding sugar. It's about embracing a powerhouse of vitamins that scaffolds a child's body against future disease.

Then there's the matter of sustainable nutrition—a concept that nudges us beyond our immediate health concerns and into the realm of environmental stewardship. As caregivers and educators, we instill not only eating habits but also values. Choosing locally sourced produce, for instance, supports local economies and reduces carbon footprints, vouching for a greener planet for those we care for.

Educating children about food origin and production opens their eyes to the impact their eating habits have worldwide. Animal-based products often have a higher ecological footprint than plant-based options. As families navigate the aisles of their grocery stores, teaching kids about this aspect of food can shape their future decisions and spur a movement towards more earth-friendly diets.

But it isn't just about what's on the plate. It's how we talk about and engage with our food. When children learn that their fish dinner may have been caught using methods that harm marine life, they begin to see their diet in a global context. They're empowered to seek alternatives that align not only with nutritional guidelines but also with a sense of global citizenship.

Moreover, the impact of food waste must be underscored. In an effort to curb this alarming trend, prompt kids to appreciate the value of their meals. Understanding the resources that go into producing their lunchbox treats can foster an appreciation that encourages them to eat mindfully and waste not.

These lessons in sustainability can go hand in hand with understanding nutritional quality. For instance, a shift towards eating more fruits and vegetables is not only beneficial for a child's health but also requires fewer resources to produce compared to animal proteins. It's a win-win. Lifelong habits of choosing plant-based options more frequently can help shape a healthier generation and planet.

And then there's water—essential for life and a critical element of sustainable food practices. Teaching children about the substantial water footprint behind myriad products heightens their awareness of conservation measures. It might just prompt them to turn the tap off a bit quicker or question the need for that almond milk carton.

Children's food choices have societal repercussions, too. Nutritional disparities exist, often reflecting socio-economic divides. By engaging young minds in discussions about food accessibility and equity, they grow with a nuanced view of the world. They become advocates for accessibility to whole, nutritious foods for everyone in their community.

It's also a matter of public health. Childhood obesity is on the rise, and diet plays a pivotal role in this trend. As we guide children to make healthier choices, we're contributing to the downward curve of this concerning trajectory. It signifies more than your child's health; it's about the collective well-being of the coming generations.

In reinforcing the value of wholesome, nutritious foods, we're implicitly teaching children to resist the alluring glow of heavily marketed, nutrient-poor options. This discernment lays a solid foundation for resisting impulsive food decisions that can lead to chronic health conditions.

Consider, too, the cultural and emotional resonance food carries. It's a conduit of heritage and comfort—a way to celebrate diversity and familial love. Yet, within this warmth, there's room for reflection. Homespun dishes steeped in tradition can be tweaked and fashioned to uphold both family history and health.

As daunting as it seems, this layering of education is an investment in a broader vision. It's about nurturing kids who are critical thinkers, environmental advocates, and guardians of their health. They'll learn to ask, "How does this food serve my body and my world?" And with every meal, they'll be casting a vote for the world they want to live in.

Ultimately, the impact of food choices is profound and multifaceted. From the immediate effects on personal health to the overarching concerns of global sustainability, every meal is a chance to educate, inspire, and shape a better future. Our role is pivotal: we can inspire a generation to be not only healthy eaters but also conscientious citizens. And every bite taken in informed mindfulness can be a small but momentous leap toward that brighter horizon.

The decisions we make at the dinner table ripple out into the world in ways we can scarcely imagine. It's a powerful form of agency that we have, and it's vital that we harness it—for our kids and for the future they will inhabit. This is the profound significance of understanding the impact of food choices.

Fostering an Eco-Friendly Approach to Eating As we navigate through the vast sea of nutritional choices for our children, it's essential to chart a course that not only ensures their health and vitality but also preserves the health of our planet. Eating with an eco-friendly approach isn't just a trend; it's a necessary shift to influence our kids' futures positively. Just as we carefully select foods to nurture their young bodies, we must tend to their food's ecological footprint.

Let's kick things off with the garden. Introducing children to the magic of planting and watching their food grow isn't just fun; it's educational. The act of gardening teaches kids about the natural cycle of life and instills an appreciation for the work that goes into producing what ends up on their plates. Whether it's a small herb garden on a windowsill or a full-fledged backyard plot, the hands-on experience connects them to the source of their sustenance and fosters respect for the environment.

Buying locally is another cardinal point on our map to eco-friendly eating. When you opt for produce from local farmers, you reduce the carbon emissions associated with long-distance food transport. Take your kids to the local farmers' market and involve them in selecting fruits and veggies. This exposes them to seasonal eating, teaches them about the local economy, and can make for an exciting family outing that links community with nutrition.

Next, consider the role of plant-based foods in your family's diet. A shift towards more fruits, vegetables, grains, and legumes, and less meat and dairy, can have a monumental effect on the environment. This doesn't necessitate a total upheaval of your dietary preferences or a leap into vegetarianism, but encouraging Meatless Mondays or plant-based snacks can significantly reduce your household's carbon footprint.

Meal planning comes to the fore when trying to avoid food waste, another cornerstone of eco-conscious eating. Plan your meals for the week with your kids and buy just what you need. This lesson in moderation not only prevents excess food from ending up in the landfill but also teaches judicious use of resources. Plus, children involved in meal planning become pickier about wasting the food they chose themselves.

Portion control is not only central to preventing overeating but also to avoiding unnecessary food waste. Teach the little ones to serve themselves age-appropriate portions or to ask for more if they're still hungry after their first serving. This way, nothing hit's the trash uneaten.

Consider your packaging practices as well. Reducing reliance on single-use plastics and opting for reusable containers, water bottles, and shopping bags teaches children to be mindful of their consumption. Demonstrating the importance of reducing, reusing, and recycling can be as simple as packing lunches in eco-friendly materials or choosing products with minimal packaging at the grocery store.

While on the topic of packaging, let's tackle the topic of processed foods. These products often come with layers of unnecessary and non-recyclable packaging, not to mention the emissions required to manufacture and transport them. Steering your family toward whole foods reduces the demand for processed foods and their environmental toll, promoting a healthier planet — and healthier children.

Conserving water is also integral to an eco-friendly diet. Educate your kids on the unseen water "ingredients" in their meals — for instance, it takes significantly more water to produce a pound of beef than a pound of grains. By choosing more water-efficient foods, you're equipping your children to make choices that support both personal and planetary hydration.

When engaging in this eco-friendly approach, be transparent with your kids about why these choices make a difference. Explain how certain foods use more resources and cause greater environmental harm than others. Ensure your discussions about sustainable eating are age-appropriate, focusing on simple concepts like "growing strong like the trees" for the younger ones and delving into more complex environmental impacts with the older children.

While discussing the effects of our food choices on the planet, teach children about carbon 'foodprints.' Explain the notion of how everything from production and processing to packaging and transport can contribute to a food item's carbon footprint. Learning this helps kids visualize the broader implications of their snack choices and the power they hold to affect change through simple actions.

Don't forget about energy use in cooking and storing food. Encouraging kids to enjoy raw snacks or foods that don't require cooking can instill habits that curb energy consumption. Similarly, understanding the energy involved in refrigeration underscores the importance of eating fresh foods that don't need long-term storage, effectively cutting down on electricity usage.

Speaking of snacks, opting for convenient pre-packaged options often contradicts eco-friendly principles. Instead, involve your kids in making homemade snacks. This can be a rewarding project that shows them the joys of making food from scratch, challenges food industry norms, and cuts back on waste.

The eco-friendly conversation is not complete without talking about the preservation of biodiversity. Educate your children about the importance of a diverse ecosystem and how varying our diet can contribute to that. Encourage them to try different foods, particularly heirloom and native species that may be less common but vitally important to environmental diversity.

Teaching kids to respect and care for the Earth through our eating choices is more than a lesson; it's a legacy. An eco-friendly approach to eating dives into the essence of teaching kids that their actions can and do make a difference. Ultimately, we're ushering in a generation of environmentally-savvy eaters who understand the symbiotic relationship between their health and the planet's. It's about nurturing a reverence for the natural world, one meal at a time.

Chapter 8:
Managing Food Allergies and Intolerances

Now that we've laid the groundwork for understanding the eco-consciousness of our kids' nutrition, let's pivot to a topic just as pivotal but more personal—navigating the often complex world of food allergies and intolerances. These are waters every parent, teacher, or caregiver might have to navigate, and doing so with grace and accuracy is vital for maintaining the health and well-being of those vibrant, energetic kids who depend on us. This chapter is your ally in decoding the signs that might point to a dietary restriction, and it arms you with strategies to ensure those restrictions don't restrict your child's zest for life. We'll tackle how to read labels with an eagle eye and understand restaurant menus with the acuity of a dietitian, all while brushing away the fog of misleading advertising tactics. What's more, we instill the confidence and knowledge in your kids to make informed choices themselves, full of empowerment and awareness. Let's confidently step into this journey of safeguarding their health, ensuring they thrive even in the face of dietary challenges.

Detecting and Dealing with Dietary Restrictions Crafting a menu that suits the kaleidoscopic diets of every child isn't merely a balancing act; it's an exercise steeped in empathy and awareness. When charting the course for healthy growth, it's paramount to identify and understand dietary restrictions that may be at play. Whether due to allergies, intolerances, or personal choices, these restrictions require vigilant attention.

First off, let's dive into detection. More often than not, dietary issues don't announce their arrival with fanfare—instead, they tend to hint at their presence subtly. For example, a child may mysteriously experience stomach upsets, skin irritations, or energy fluctuations that seem disconnected from their usual health. Professionals and caretakers need to become detectives, using clues from these reactions to determine whether food might be the culprit. A comprehensive food journal, documenting everything a child eats, can be the magnifying glass that brings these clues into focus.

If your spidey-senses are tingling, it may be time to bring in the experts for confirmation. A visit to the allergist or gastroenterologist can clarify the situation and ensure that any dietary changes you contemplate are grounded in medical advice, not just assumption. These visits aren't just about testing; they're about equipping you and the child with an understanding of the body's needs and how to meet them safely.

Once a dietary restriction is confirmed, clear communication becomes your best ally. This involves explicating what the child can and can't eat, why this is so, and establishing a plan. It's essential that the child feels included in this conversation—after all, it's their body, and understanding their needs lays the groundwork for self-sufficiency as they grow.

Dealing with dietary restrictions takes vigilance, particularly in communal settings such as schools or birthday parties. It's crucial to communicate a child's dietary needs to educators and other parents. Providing them with specifics as well as simple alternatives can prevent accidental exposure and make the child feel included, not excluded, from group activities.

Meal planning for children with dietary restrictions necessitates creativity. Instead of focusing on what's off-limits, shine a light on the diverse array of foods that are available and compatible. This positive framing can help children to feel less restricted and more excited about their options.

When you're juggling dietary restrictions, knowledge of substitutions becomes your secret weapon. Nut butters can replace dairy butters in baking. Zoodles can stand in for pasta for gluten-free diets. A well-stocked pantry with these alternative ingredients means you're always ready to whip up a meal that's both nutritious and restriction-friendly.

Learning how to read labels is an important skill for anyone managing dietary restrictions. Encourage older children to read the labels themselves, turning it into a fun and educational exercise. This practice not only builds independence but also reinforces the importance of knowing what goes into their bodies.

Trust is essential when managing a child's dietary restrictions, but so is teaching them to ask the important questions when you're not there to advocate for them. Practice scenarios where they might need to verify ingredients, so they feel confident to do so in real-life situations.

Don't overlook the emotional dimension of dietary restrictions. Food is often the center of social interactions, and feeling different can be challenging for a child. Heal potential emotional wounds with open dialogues about how it's okay to have different needs and that diversity is a strength, not a weakness.

When you find yourself at a loss or in need of inspiration, turn to communities—both virtual and real—where others share similar experiences. These platforms can offer support, recipes, and personal stories that spotlight the successful navigation of dietary restrictions. Children can even find peers who are like them, which might make their unique eating patterns feel more normal and accepted.

Don't forget to celebrate the wins. Found a great allergy-friendly recipe that the whole family loves? Made it through a party without any hiccups? These victories, big or small, should be acknowledged and cherished. They reinforce the reality that while dietary restrictions may require careful thought and planning, they need not diminish the joy of eating and discovery.

Educating yourself and staying current with the latest information about food allergies and intolerances is imperative. Regulations change, as do the understanding and management of dietary restrictions. Remaining informed means you can provide the best care and make the most informed choices for the child's well-being.

Institutions such as schools and camps are increasingly aware of the need to accommodate dietary restrictions. Collaborate with them to ensure they have policies in place that enable children with dietary needs to participate fully and safely. Encourage a culture of inclusiveness that extends to the cafeteria menu and classroom snack times.

Ultimately, detecting and dealing with dietary restrictions in children isn't just about managing what they eat—it's about nurturing resilience, fostering independence, and instilling a sense of normalcy despite those restrictions. It's about teaching them that while they have to navigate their world a little differently, it's still a world full of flavor, community, and joy.

Keeping Kids Safe and Well-Nourished in the context of managing food allergies and intolerances is a task that can seem daunting at first. It's all about creating an environment where kids can thrive, even with dietary restrictions. As we navigate this terrain, the essential goal is to arm ourselves—and our children—with the knowledge and skills they need to make healthy choices that keep them safe and their bodies nourished.

It's critical to recognize that food allergies and sensitivities can significantly impact a child's quality of life. This is where understanding comes into play. A deep understanding of your child's unique needs is the first step towards ensuring their safety and well-being. This means knowing not only which foods to avoid but also how to find nutritious and enjoyable alternatives that maintain a balanced diet.

Education is your ally. Teaching kids about their allergies in an age-appropriate manner helps them understand the risks and the importance of reading labels and asking questions. It's empowering for a child to feel in control of their situation; it can boost their confidence and help them feel less alienated in social situations involving food.

Communication is key, not only with your child but also with others who play a role in their day-to-day life, such as teachers, babysitters, and parents of their friends. Transparent dialogues about what food safety means for your child are essential. This ensures that everyone on your child's support team is on the same page and can recognize and respond to an allergic reaction if necessary.

Reading labels should be second nature to you and your child. But it's more than just looking for the obvious allergens; it's about being able to decipher less obvious ingredients that could pose a threat. We're not just talking about an academic exercise. It's a real-life skill that can protect your child's health.

Considering the nutritional content of allergen-free products is important. Sometimes, products made to be free of common allergens may lack essential nutrients. Therefore, striking a balance is crucial. Opting for whole foods, whenever possible, and supplementing the diet wisely to make up for any nutritional deficiencies is a strategy that works.

Meal planning is incredibly beneficial when it comes to keeping allergic children safe and well-nourished. Planning meals ensures that you're prepared with safe options that contribute to a balanced diet. You're architecting a diverse menu that keeps your child interested in eating while meeting all their dietary needs.

Let's not overlook the role of creativity in the kitchen. Coming up with allergen-free dishes that are both nutritious and exciting can make all the difference. It transforms mealtime from a potential source of anxiety to an enjoyable experience. Allergen-free doesn't have to mean taste-free or fun-free.

Build a network. Connecting with other parents and caregivers who are in the same boat can offer a treasure trove of resources, from recipes to coping strategies. Support groups can be a beautiful place to share stories and solutions, helping you navigate this journey with less stress and more success.

Don't forget about dining out. While it can be more challenging, it's not impossible. It's about equipping your child with the ability to ask the right questions and choose safely when eating at a restaurant. Talking to chefs and staff about your child's needs is part of the new normal, and many are happy to accommodate.

Nutrient supplementation may sometimes be necessary, but it should always be handled with care. Consulting with a healthcare provider to understand which supplements, if any, your child may need can ensure they're getting a well-rounded arsenal of nutrients required for growth and development.

Part of keeping kids safe is also teaching them to advocate for themselves. As they grow older, they'll need to make food choices without your direct supervision. Equip them with the confidence and knowledge to make these decisions responsibly by role-playing different scenarios and discussing potential outcomes.

Schools are another arena where safety and nourishment are of paramount importance. Work with school administrators to ensure that appropriate measures are in place—from allergen-free zones to staff trained in recognizing and treating allergic reactions. Knowing that their school environment is safe can greatly ease anxiety for both children and parents.

Finally, don't ignore the emotional and psychological impact that food allergies can have on a child. Offering emotional support and understanding can be just as important as managing the physical aspects of their diet. Celebrate the wins, big or small, and stay optimistic. Children pick up on this energy and it can help them feel more positive about their dietary journey.

With diligence, care, and creativity, you can craft a safe and satisfying dietary life for your child, even within the bounds of food allergies and intolerances. It's about empowerment, education, and a little bit of elbow grease in the kitchen. Together, you can navigate this path, ensuring that your child's well-being is the top priority and demonstrating that a fulfilling life doesn't have to be compromised by dietary restrictions.

Reading Labels and Restaurant Menus is a vital skill in fostering heathy eating habits among children. Just as we learned in earlier sections about establishing a positive food environment and designing well-balanced meals, it's equally important to navigate the world of food outside the home. Considering how labels and menus can either be informative or misleading, understanding them is crucial for making informed dietary choices.

Think of a food label as a mini encyclopedia of what's inside the package. It gives information about nutrients, ingredients, and more. Start by looking at the serving size, which can be surprisingly smaller than you might expect. Teach your kids that if a container has more than one serving, they need to multiply the nutritional information on the label by the number of servings they consume to get an accurate picture.

Calories are another important aspect of the label, but remember, they're not the only thing that counts. The quality and source of these calories matter a lot. Introduce the concept that calories from whole foods like fruits and vegetables are far better than calories from sugary snacks. But do so in a way that eschews demonizing foods, instead, promote balance and informed decisions.

When it comes to nutrients, there are some you want less of, and others you want more. Saturated fats, trans fats, cholesterol, and sodium are best consumed in moderation. On the other hand, dietary fiber, vitamin D, calcium, iron, and potassium are nutrients to encourage. Use the label to guide kids towards these smarter choices.

Sugar content warrants special attention, especially added sugars. These are not the naturally occurring sugars found in dairy and fruit but are added during processing. Encourage your little ones to recognize and prefer foods with low added sugars, for their overall health and development.

While labels provide a wealth of information, they can also be tricky. Watch out for serving sizes that are unrealistic or claims that may not tell the whole story — like "low fat" which might mean "high in sugar." Teach kids to be detectives, looking beyond the flashy claims on the front of the package to the facts on the back.

Ingredients lists are another insightful area. They are ordered by quantity, from most to least. This is a great place to spot additives, preservatives, and artificial colors, which are best to avoid. Encourage kids to spot whole foods in the ingredient list and understand that shorter lists often indicate less processed foods.

Now, let's translate this knowledge to restaurant menus, which don't often come with detailed nutritional information. However, that doesn't mean you're flying blind. Opt for dishes with a lot of vegetables, lean proteins, and whole grains. When in doubt, it's perfectly alright to ask the server about how a dish is prepared or to request modifications like dressing on the side.

Portion sizes at restaurants can be misleading, just like on food labels. They are often much larger than what is recommended for a single serving. Splitting a meal or taking some home can be a smart way to manage this reality. Instill this habit in children by encouraging them to listen to their hunger signals and stop eating when they are full, not when the plate is empty.

Educate children on the topic of "choice architecture" right there on the menu. Items in a box, with pictures, or at the top of a list are designed to catch their eye. They may not always align with the healthiest options, so it's important to choose deliberately and not just follow the visual cues.

Don't shy away from discussing how restaurants often optimize the taste of their dishes with extra sugar, salt, or fat — far more than we might use at home. This doesn't mean dining out is a no-go, but it's about making better choices, such as grilled instead of fried options or skipping the sugary soda in favor of water.

If there's an option for a children's menu, it often contains highly processed, fried, and sugary options. Instead, focus on the main menu where there are opportunities to share healthier dishes. This also models the idea that kids don't need a separate menu to eat healthily; they too can enjoy a variety of foods.

There's also a place for flexibility and enjoyment. Kids should learn that eating out can include special treats or less frequent foods, but it's about the context within their overall diet. A slice of cake to celebrate a birthday at a restaurant is a delightful part of life, as long as it's not an everyday choice.

In our journey towards fostering healthy eating in kids, it's essential to teach them to discern the good from the not-so-good. Equip them with the knowledge to understand food labels and make smarter choices in restaurants. This way, whether they're reaching for a snack at the grocery store or ordering a meal out, they're empowered to choose with health in mind.

Remember that kids are curious and capable learners. When we take the time to explore labels and menus with them, ask questions, and make it a learning experience, we're not just feeding them for a day — we're teaching them nutritional habits for a lifetime. So let's embrace this role as their guide, helping them to navigate the vast sea of dietary choices with confidence and knowledge.

Unpacking Advertising Tactics As we navigate the intricate world of dietary restrictions, allergies, and reading labels, it's crucial to also equip ourselves and our kids with the ability to decode the often-cunning world of food advertising. It's a battleground where psychology meets creativity, and understanding these tactics helps us foster healthier eating habits in youngsters. This section delves deep into the methods employed by advertisers to attract the attention and loyalty of children and how we can educate our children to see beyond the façade.

Firstly, let's talk about the allure of bright colors and characters. Whether it's a cartoon mascot or the vivid rainbow shades on a cereal box, these strategies are anything but random. They're meticulously designed to catch the eye of the youngest consumers, tapping into their love for animated shows and playful imagery. Teaching kids to recognize these characters and colors as marketing tools can help them become more discerning consumers.

Another widely used tactic is the promise of fun and toys. Fast food chains often entice children with the latest toy from popular movie franchises, using these freebies as bait to sell their meal options.

It's not just meals—snack and cereal manufacturers include toys, stickers, or games inside or on their packaging, making the product more desirable. When children understand that the real value lies in the nutrients they consume, not the trinkets that come with them, they're better equipped to make healthier choices.

Social proof plays a significant role in advertising to children, with ads frequently showing groups of kids having a blast while indulging in the advertised product. Peer influence is powerful, and when it seems like everyone else is enjoying a certain snack, a child might feel left out if they don't partake. It's crucial to have conversations with kids about the importance of good nutrition over following the crowd.

Endorsements from celebrities or athletes can create an aura of desirability around products. Having a sports star claim that a sugar-laden sports drink is to thank for their performance may compel kids to believe that's their ticket to athleticism. Instilling a critical mindset and discussing the truth behind advertising claims is key to not getting swept up by celebrity influence.

Fostering skepticism is beneficial when it comes to extravagant health claims. Advertisers often label foods as "natural" or packed with vitamins to create a health halo that isn't always fully justified. It's essential to help children understand these labels and to look closer at ingredient lists to see if the claims stand up to scrutiny.

Noise and action are staples of ads targeting children because they mimic the high energy and chaos that kids find entertaining. Commercials for sugary cereals or snacks are often fast-paced, loud, and filled with action-packed scenarios which can subliminally link excitement with the product. Remind youngsters that true excitement comes from playing and interacting, not from what's inside a brightly colored box.

Creating a sense of urgency can influence immediate desire. "Limited time offers" or items that claim to be "selling out fast" can prompt a fear of missing out. Discussing with children that good food doesn't need to be bought in a rush can instill patience and thoughtfulness in their consumption habits.

The language in advertising is also tailored to charm young ears with phrases like "mega blast flavors" or "power-packed punch". This clever wording can make a regular snack sound extraordinary. Encourage kids to find the real 'power' in foods; that is, their nutritional value and how they fuel the body.

Interactive websites and advertising games, known as 'advergames', blur the line between play and product promotion. These games are often full of brand imagery and product placement, embedding brand loyalty at a young age. Show children how real games and activities are infinitely more enriching for their minds and bodies.

Celebratory tie-ins with holidays and events can make certain foods seem essential for a good time. From Halloween candy to Christmas cookies, ads can make it seem like these treats are an integral part of the festivities. Cultivating family traditions that focus on togetherness rather than food can help counter this effect.

Lastly, through product placement in movies and TV shows, food and beverage brands often have characters use or discuss their products within the storyline. This casual integration makes the consumption of these products appear normal and desirable. It's important for kids to learn the difference between storytelling and advertising within their favorite shows.

Understanding advertising tactics is about more than just resisting the constant barrage of marketing - it's about empowering children to make informed, healthy choices even in the face of persuasive messaging. This critical awareness ensures that they are equipped to navigate an environment saturated with appeals for their attention and ultimately their appetites.

As adults, we have a responsibility to not only talk about these tactics but to also model behavior that reflects our teachings. When children see us making informed choices, questioning marketing claims, laughing at the absurdity of some advertisements, and valuing nutrition over gimmicks, they're more likely to emulate these attitudes. It's not just about telling them, it's about showing them how to live a life less influenced by the smoke and mirrors of advertising.

Remember that our role is to be advocates for our children's health. By unpacking the complexities of advertising, we are equipping them with the critical thinking skills necessary to thrive in a consumer-centric world. It's not just about saying no to the unhealthy options; it's about fostering an understanding that leads to a lifetime of wise and mindful eating choices.

Building this comprehensive awareness is not an overnight task. It's an ongoing conversation that evolves as kids grow and as advertising tactics change. Let's commit to staying informed so we can continue to guide the next generation in making food choices that are as much about their well-being as they are about enjoyment.

Empowering Kids to Make Informed Choices As we delve deeper into the dynamic world of guiding kids towards healthier eating, it's crucial to understand how empowerment plays a key role. Empowering our children means giving them the knowledge and confidence to make choices that are beneficial for their health and wellbeing. This chapter highlights ways we can equip our children with the skills they need to navigate the complex food landscape before them.

First, let's talk about the power of information. Providing children with age-appropriate knowledge about nutrition helps demystify food choices. When kids learn what vitamins and minerals do for their bodies, they begin to see food as more than just something that tastes good—it's fuel, a provider of energy, and a means to grow stronger.

When kids have the tools to understand why some foods are eaten sparingly while others can be enjoyed more freely, they're more likely to make sound decisions. This isn't about drilling dietary guidelines into their heads, but rather it's about engaging them in conversations about why certain foods can make them feel vibrant and active, while others might leave them feeling sluggish.

Teaching kids to read labels is another component of empowering them. Show them the ropes — the realities of sugar content, the presence of additives, and the importance of whole food ingredients. By doing this, you're not only informing them, you're fostering critical thinking skills that they'll use in all areas of their lives.

Another effective strategy is involving children in meal planning and grocery shopping. This not only makes them feel valued and responsible, but also gives them practical experience. They can learn to make healthy choices by picking out fresh produce or comparing the nutrition of different products.

Let's not shy away from discussing how marketing influences food choices. Kids are bombarded with advertisements for all sorts of products, many of which are far from healthy. By educating them on advertising tactics, we can prepare them to recognize and resist manipulative marketing ploys. This awareness fosters a discerning mindset that prioritizes their health and needs over catchy slogans and flashy packaging.

Children often feel empowered when they have autonomy. Allowing them to make their own food choices within a set of healthy options can instill a sense of independence. This could be as simple as letting them pick between carrots and cucumbers for a snack or choosing the fruit for a smoothie. Small choices add up to big confidence.

Discussing the environmental impact of food choices is also a form of empowerment. When children understand that they can help the planet by what they put on their plate, it instills an early sense of stewardship. Choices like opting for locally sourced vegetables or less meat can become compelling ways for kids to feel they're making a difference.

Role-playing can be an enjoyable and informative tool. Through role-playing scenarios, kids can practice how to choose healthy options when dining out or how to courteously decline foods they're allergic to or just prefer not to eat. Rehearsing these situations helps reduce anxiety and builds assertiveness.

What about those times when choices are limited, such as at a school cafeteria or a friend's house? Teaching kids to do the best they can with available options encourages adaptability and resilience. They can learn to choose the healthiest item on a menu or to balance a less nutritious meal with healthier choices later in the day.

Encouragement and praise are profound motivators. As kids practice making informed choices, acknowledging their efforts and good decisions reinforces their behavior. Positive feedback nurtures their decision-making skills and boosts their confidence to continue making healthy choices.

Empowerment also comes from understanding that making the 'less healthy' choice occasionally is okay, as long as it's balanced with nutritious foods most of the time. Helping kids manage these situations without guilt supports a healthy relationship with food and prevents it from becoming a source of stress or negativity.

As we approach the conclusion of this empowering chapter, remember that informed food choices are just one aspect of a healthy lifestyle for kids. We must not forget the synergy between a well-balanced diet, physical activity, and mental health. Each is a puzzle piece in the grand scheme of a child's wellbeing.

In summary, empowering kids to make informed choices about their food involves education, experience, critical thinking, and encouragement. It's about creating an environment where children are taught to value nutrition, understand the implications of their food choices, and feel confident in their ability to choose well—for their health, the environment, and ultimately, their futures.

As parents and caregivers, let's take pride in knowing that each lesson we impart, and each choice we help our children make, is a step toward their autonomy and lifelong well-being. With every seed of knowledge planted, we're empowering a generation of mindful eaters, ready to make informed choices for a lifetime of health and satisfaction.

Chapter 9:
The Snack Conundrum

We've ventured through the meandering roads of nutrition, picked up strategies to handle even the most resolute picky eater, and discussed how to maintain balance and safety with dietary restrictions. Now, let's set our sights on a stumbling block that trips up many—the snack conundrum. Children hunger for snacks, but not all nibbles are created equal. It's tempting to yield to the convenience of processed options, yet we know they often pack a sugary punch and lack nutrient density. So how do we pivot towards whole foods that fulfill and excite those tiny tummies? Think of snacks as mini-meals; they are opportunities to fuel growing bodies and infuse an extra dose of vitamins and minerals. By being intentional about our snack selection, we're not just quelling hunger, we're contributing to the intricate mosaic of a child's health. With a dash of creativity, a pinch of planning, we can transform snack time into a vibrant, health-boosting segment of the day. One that competes with the alluring world of shiny, packaged temptations. And remember, snacks don't have to be dull or time-consuming; with an arsenal of quick, appealing, and nutritious ideas, they can be convenient, visually enticing, and deliciously satisfying.

Choosing Whole Foods Over Processed Snacks In previous chapters, we've laid down the fundamental roles of macronutrients, a multitude of vitamins and minerals deemed essential for our little ones, and methods to create an environment that promotes healthy eating.

As we journey further, the spotlight now falls on the significant benefits of selecting whole foods over processed snacks, a choice that not only influences a child's current health but also sets the foundation for their dietary patterns in the future.

Let's begin with an undeniable premise: kids love to snack. It's a natural part of their day, providing an energy boost and satisfying hunger between meals. But not all snacks are created equal. The convenience of processed snacks can be tempting; they're often designed to be irresistibly tasty and easy to grab on the go. However, they frequently lack nutritional value and are packed with added sugars, sodium, and unhealthy fats.

To steer children towards better health, one of the most powerful choices we can make is to choose whole foods as snacks. Whole foods are those that have been processed or refined as little as possible, and are free from additives or other artificial substances. They're closer to their natural form, brimming with essential nutrients that growing bodies need.

Whole foods come as single-ingredient treasures like fruits, nuts, and vegetables. They are nutrient-dense, which means they're packed with vitamins, minerals, fiber, and other beneficial compounds. For instance, an apple is much more than just a sweet treat. It's a complex, fibrous package that delivers vitamin C, potassium, and various phytonutrients that can contribute to overall health.

The focus on whole foods is also a step back to basics, showcasing the flavors, textures, and joys of eating food as nature provides. Encouraging kids to enjoy a handful of almonds or carrot sticks with hummus instead of a bag of chips can challenge their palates and help them appreciate the natural taste of food, without the need for heavy processing or additives.

One argument against whole foods is the convenience factor. Sure, opening a packet of cookies takes seconds, while washing and slicing an apple might take a couple of minutes more. But think of these extra minutes as an investment in your child's lifelong health. The additional effort teaches them the importance of self-care and setting aside time to nourish their body properly.

Making the switch to whole foods also presents an opportunity to introduce children to the concept of mindfulness when it comes to eating. Mindfulness encourages being fully present and engaged in the eating experience, which can lead to better digestion and greater satisfaction with the foods consumed. A fresh peach, with its juicy burst of flavor, can become a sensory delight, urging kids to eat more slowly and savor every bite.

A significant factor in promoting whole foods is the example set by parents and caregivers. When children see the adults in their lives opting for real, unprocessed foods, they're more likely to follow suit. It's much easier to get kids excited about snacking on whole foods when they see those they look up to doing the same.

Offering a variety of whole food snacks can also help prevent flavor fatigue and keep children's interest piqued. Mix it up with seasonal fruits and vegetables, a rotation of nuts and seeds, and even some whole grains like popcorn without added artificial flavors or excess salt. Variety not only keeps it fun but ensures a wider range of nutrients is consumed.

Equally important is involving kids in the selection process of whole food snacks. Take them along when shopping for groceries and let them pick out what looks good to them. This autonomy can be incredibly empowering and can inspire more enthusiasm for snacking on whole foods.

But we can go even further. Education is essential, and explaining why whole foods are a better choice can make a significant difference. Discussing the benefits of the nutrients found in these foods and how they help kids grow, learn, and play can foster an understanding that goes beyond the simple act of eating.

Preparing whole food snacks can also be a bonding activity. Kids are more likely to eat what they've helped make. Simple tasks like washing fruits, peeling oranges, or cutting vegetables (with supervision) are not just educational; they're steps on the road toward independence and self-reliance in healthy eating.

While making the switch, remember that balance is key. The occasional processed snack won't derail a healthy diet, but the goal is to ensure such snacks do not become the default. Creating an environment where whole food snacks are the standard sets the tone for balanced eating habits.

In the end, the decision to select whole foods over processed snacks isn't just about the single snack moment—it's about shaping palate preferences, nutrition education, and a larger health-conscious lifestyle. Teaching kids to reach for an orange instead of orange-flavored candy is a subtle shift that reverberates through their lives, echoing into adulthood with profound health benefits.

As the snack conundrum unravels, we arrive at the understanding that our decisions are powerful. They carry the weight to change the trajectory of our children's health and well-being. Embracing whole foods over processed snacks arms children with an arsenal of nutrients vital for their abundant energy and growth. It is one of the purest forms of care that we, as parents and caregivers, can provide—a legacy of health, one snack at a time.

Creative and Appealing Snack Ideas Let's dive into the delicious world of snacks that are sure to catch the attention of children while also nurturing their growing bodies. Often, it's the colorful and fun presentation that wins over kids' hearts and palates. Think rainbow fruit skewers or a platter of veggies arranged in the shape of their favorite animal. It's about making healthy snacks as visually appealing as they are tasty.

Have you ever seen the spark in a child's eyes when they spot a treat that's both whimsical and flavorful? Let's harness that enthusiasm with snacks that are as nutritious as they are delightful. Imagine transforming ordinary apple slices into 'apple donuts' topped with almond butter and a sprinkle of granola. It's a simple flip that combines fruit with protein and fiber without compromising on the fun factor.

Another game-changer in the snacking department is blending colorful smoothies. They're like sippable rainbows, each color bursting with vitamins and minerals. A mix of leafy greens, frozen berries, and a banana can become an 'Incredible Hulk' smoothie; not only does it look cool, but it also sneaks in those veggies in the tastiest way possible.

For an energizing snack that packs a protein punch, think mini kabobs. Skewer cubes of cheese, cherry tomatoes, and whole-grain bread, and you've created a snack that covers several food groups. It's a hands-on eating experience that's mess-free and perfectly portioned for little hands.

On to the sweeter side, yogurt can be the canvas for an array of toppings. You can layer yogurt with pureed fruit to create beautiful parfaits or freeze them to make homemade frozen yogurt pops. They're delightful to look at and guilt-free to enjoy. Plus, they're an excellent way for kids to get their probiotics.

Nuts and seeds can be tough sells on their own, but when they're part of a homemade trail mix with a few dark chocolate chips and dried fruit, they become an irresistible snack. It's a tactful way to introduce healthy fats and proteins into a child's diet while still satisfying their cravings for something sweet and crunchy.

For those times when convenience is key, consider whole grain crackers paired with fun dips like hummus or guacamole. Arranging these on a plate with a mix of colors and shapes can turn a simple snack into an interactive and joyful experience. Plus, it encourages kids to explore different flavors and textures.

Don't overlook the power of a good ol' peanut butter and banana sandwich, with a twist. Use a cookie cutter to turn it into stars, hearts, or even dinosaurs. These playful shapes aren't just cute; they make the whole eating process a memorable adventure for kids.

Puffed rice cakes can be the basis for snack-sized pizzas. Let kids add their choice of toppings, such as tomato sauce, shredded cheese, and a mix of vegetables. This not only tantalizes their taste buds but also gets them involved in the snack-making process, encouraging a hands-on approach to healthy eating.

For a savory snack with a crunch, roasted chickpeas are a fabulous choice. Season them with a kid-friendly spice mix, and they'll be asking for more. This legume is loaded with protein and fiber, making it an excellent snack for sustained energy throughout the day.

When the weather heats up, nothing beats homemade ice pops. By blending fruits and even vegetables with a little juice and freezing them in molds, you can create a cold treat that's full of nutrients. They're a fabulous way to hydrate and cool down after active play.

Another wonderful idea is to use whole-grain tortillas as a base for creating rolls or wraps. Fill them with combinations of turkey, lettuce, cheese, or even peanut butter and jelly. Rolled up and sliced into bite-sized pieces, they're fun to eat and filled with good-for-you ingredients.

Now, if you're aiming for something a little more indulgent yet still within the realm of healthy, dark chocolate-dipped fruit might be the ticket. Bananas, strawberries, or even oranges dipped in a thin layer of dark chocolate provide antioxidants without going overboard on sugar.

Last but not least, don't forget about the power of popcorn. When it's air-popped and lightly seasoned, it's a whole-grain snack that can easily become a favorite. It's perfect for movie nights or as a handy snack that kids can help prepare.

Within these creative ideas lies a symphony of flavors and nutrients, waiting to enchant children and instill a love for wholesome, healthy snacks. Keep in mind that the key to success is variety, balance, and a touch of playfulness—children are more likely to reach for snacks that tickle their imagination as well as their taste buds.

Chapter 10:
Hydration and Health

As we leave behind the intricate world of macronutrients and smart snacking, it's time we soak up the essentials of hydration and its pivotal role in our children's health. Let's face it, water may not have the flashiness of flavored drinks, but it's the unsung hero keeping our little ones energized, focused, and growing strong. Every cell, every tissue, and every system in their bustling young bodies relies on water to function smoothly. Knowing that, we've got a responsibility to turn the tide against sugary drinks while navigating toward nourishing hydration habits. It's about recognizing thirst signals, setting a stellar example, and maybe, just once in a while, cutting loose with a splashy water fight on a hot afternoon. Encouraging water intake isn't just about quenching thirst, it's about laying the foundation for a lifetime of good health. So, let's pour our efforts into making water the beverage of choice, keeping our kids vibrant, alert, and ready for every playful challenge life tosses their way.

Why Water is Essential In crafting a blueprint for healthy eating and thriving young lives, water stands out as a pillar of well-being that's often overlooked. It's a simple compound, H2O, yet its benefits are vast and vital for the developing bodies of children. As caregivers and educators, our task is to spotlight water not just as a mere thirst-quencher but as an essential nutrient that carries monumental importance in the daily diet of children.

Think of a child's body as an exuberant stream of energy. Just as streams require a steady flow of water to sustain the ecosystem, our kids need water to fuel their biological intricacies. It's a critical component of bodily functions, facilitating digestion, absorption of nutrients, and waste removal. Diving into the cells, tissues, and organs of young ones, we uncover that water is the medium where all life processes occur, underscoring its significance.

Water also regulates body temperature, a function that's especially crucial for active kids. Whether they're conquering the jungle gym or engaging in team sports, their bodies generate heat. Water aids in dissipating this heat through perspiration, preventing overheating and maintaining a safe internal environment. It's clear then, that water isn't simply about quenching thirst—it's a built-in cooling system.

As children grow, their brains develop at a rapid pace, calling for optimal hydration. Adequate water intake is linked to improved cognitive function, better concentration, and alertness. It's like oil to a machine—essential for peak performance. Without it, the risk of lethargy, confusion, and inattention rises, potential barriers to learning and developmental progress.

But it's not just about drinking water when the mind signals thirst. By then, the body may already be in a state of dehydration. It's critical to promote regular sipping throughout the day to maintain hydration before thirst kicks in. This way, their bodies never have to experience the setback of dehydration.

Furthermore, water plays a role in maintaining a healthy weight. It's a natural appetite suppressant, free of calories, sugars, and additives found in many other beverages marketed towards children. Encouraging water over sugary drinks can help instill habits that steer clear of empty calories and potential weight issues.

Speaking of dental health, water—particularly when it's fluoridated—supports strong teeth formation and helps combat tooth decay. It's a mighty ally in the battle against cavities, and unlike those sweetened beverages, it doesn't contribute to dental erosion. Promoting water not only quenches thirst but also conserves those precious smiles.

For athletic or simply active kids, water replenishes the fluids lost through sweat. It's the source of vitality needed to maintain endurance and prevent the adverse effects of dehydration, such as muscle cramps and fatigue. By staying hydrated, children can play, learn, and grow with fewer interruptions.

Hydration isn't something that we should leave to chance or serendipity. It's a habit to be woven into the fabric of daily life, a norm to be modeled by parents and educators alike. By creating a water-friendly environment, we send the message that water is just as important as the foods on their plates.

So, what does establishing a good hydration habit look like? It starts with making water accessible. Keep it in plain sight, offer it at meals and snacks, and discuss its importance. Equip kids with their water bottles and praise them for refueling their tanks. It's about celebrating water, not as a mundane necessity but as the elixir of life.

When it comes to mealtimes, water should be the drink of choice. It complements the nutrients found in healthy foods, facilitating their journey around the body. It's the unsung hero of a balanced meal, an enabler of the body's symphonic metabolic processes.

It's also worth noting that not all children's water needs are the same—active kids, those living in hot climates, or who are ill with fever or gastrointestinal symptoms may need more. It's important to adjust intake accordingly and pay heed to these shifting requirements to ensure their tanks are well topped off for optimal health and growth.

Cutting through the ocean of beverage options, water stands out as the beacon of hydration. It's nature's solution to many of the dietary challenges children face today. It's about nudging our kids to listen to their bodies and use water as their first tool in maintaining balance and wellness.

Finally, in addressing hydration, we're fostering a lifelong habit that sets children on a path to continuous health. The totality of water's role in the growth, development, and daily performance of children can't be overstated. It's the foundation for a vibrant childhood and a thriving life, and we're the stewards guiding our kids toward that well-hydrated future.

As we continue our journey through this book, remember the simplicity and power of water. It's not just about the food on the plate—it's equally about the water in the glass alongside it. Let's endeavor to keep our children's hydration a top priority as we build upon their nutritional wellness, one sip at a time.

Limiting Sugary Drinks and Encouraging Water Intake As we've immersed ourselves in the essence of a healthy diet for children, we've touched on macronutrients, the might of minerals, and the vitality of various vitamins. Moving deeper into our hydration chapter, we're focusing on a critical component of youth nutrition: the liquid landscape. Picking up the sippy cup where we left off, let's navigate the sugary seas, steering our kids towards more salubrious shores.

Sugary drinks are akin to trojan horses in children's diets, laden with empty calories and a lack of nutrients, yet often welcomed with open arms due to their tantalizing taste. Be it soda, juice, sports drinks, or flavored milk, what often seems like a harmless treat can, over time, accumulate unwanted effects on body weight and dental health. Therefore, we've got our work cut out for us in mitigating these sweet sips.

The first step is understanding why it's critical to limit these liquid sugars. Studies have linked heavy consumption of sweetened beverages to obesity, type 2 diabetes, and even heart disease later in life. While one drink won't tip the scales, habitual intake can set a pattern that's tough to break. Let's be mindful that every drop counts.

Now, it's about striking a balance. Discouraging sugary drinks doesn't mean we declare an outright ban. Encouragement always trumps enforcement. Reserve these drinks for special occasions, reducing their status from staple to rarity. This subtle shift reinforces the idea that these are treats, not everyday necessities.

For those moments when water does not entertain the palates of our little ones, we can introduce healthier alternatives. Try infusing water with fruits like berries or citrus slices for a touch of natural sweetness. Unsweetened teas can also be a flavorful escape from monotony, and the making of them can be a sensory adventure for children, as they watch the colors diffuse and taste the subtle flavors.

Empowering children with knowledge about what they're drinking contributes to informed decisions. Explain how water is a powerful potion for their bodies, aiding every function from digestion to cognition. Turn hydration into a science lesson about the human body, and let their curiosity lead them to choose the superior drink— H2O.

One cannot overlook the role modeling plays in encouraging healthy hydration habits. If they see adults opting for water, they're more inclined to follow suit. Keep water easily accessible, in fun bottles or cups that are solely theirs, reinforcing ownership and choice in the matter of hydration.

Schools, too, should be sanctuaries of healthful habits. Advocate for accessible water stations and policies that limit the availability of sugary drinks within school grounds. When water becomes the norm, children adapt with surprising ease.

Interestingly, gamification can go a long way in enticing children to drink more water. Track their intake with stickers or a chart for a visual representation of their accomplishment. Assign rewards for consistent hydration practices, not based on the quantity per se, but on the regularity of their water consumption.

Making water intake a family challenge can also stoke the fires of friendly competition. Who reached for water first thing in the morning? Who refilled their bottle the most? Shared objectives foster unity and spur everyone on to better health.

Furthermore, when planning outings or packing lunches, preempt the temptation to purchase sugary drinks by bringing along filled water bottles. Make it a ritual that going out equals taking water along. This simple act instills the habit of healthy hydration outside the home.

Menus at home should also undergo a liquid transformation. During meals, make water the main beverage on the table. Encourage sips between bites, which not only aids in hydration but also slows down eating, allowing the body to register fullness more accurately.

Lastly, remember the power of praise. When children choose water over a sweetened drink, commend their choice. Positive reinforcement nurtures self-esteem and reinforces good decision-making for the future.

Laying the keel for lifelong hydration habits is no fleeting endeavor. It calls for patience, creativity, and consistency. As we imbibe these practices within our homes and communities, we pave the way for children to emerge as healthier, more informed, and empowered consumers. Let's raise a glass to that—a glass brimming with pure water, the elixir of life.

Chapter 11:
Navigating School Cafeterias and Social Settings

As we pivot from the importance of hydration, we dive into the bustling world of school cafeterias and the dynamics of social gatherings—arenas where children's nutritional choices are put to the test. Venturing through these communal spaces, we'll explore tactics to help kids make mindful food selections amidst an array of less-than-nutritious temptations. These settings are often where peer influence and enticing presentations can lead even the most health-conscious child astray. Empowerment is key; let's equip our youngsters with the know-how to navigate these nutritional minefields confidently, balancing the enjoyment of occasional treats with maintaining a diet rich in wholesome sustenance. In this chapter, we'll address how to gracefully manage the festive allure of birthday parties and the casual comfort of sleepovers, ensuring our children can partake in the joy of childhood without compromising on their well-being.

School Lunches: Nutrition vs. Appeal As we turn the pages from understanding the basics of nutrition and the role of parents in shaping their children's eating habits, let's delve into an environment that heavily influences what our little ones consume - the school cafeteria. This is the battlefield where nutrition often meets its foe: the appeal of less healthy options.

School lunches stand at the crossroads of health education and real-life choices, and we must tackle head-on the challenges they present. It's here that the principles taught at home are put to the test, where carrots can become less shiny in the light of cheese-drenched nachos or the humble apple less tempting beside a bag of chips.

Understandably, our kids are wired to crave the salt, sugar, and fats that processed foods deliver in abundance. But remember, healthy lunches aren't just about the nutrients – they're about creating meals kids actually want to eat. It's paramount to strike a balance, ensuring meals are as appealing to the taste buds and eyes as they are nourishing to the body.

So how do we navigate this tightrope? First, we have to consider what kids love. Familiarity and fun play crucial roles. Introducing new veggies? Pair them with a beloved dip. Whole grains can be a hard sell, but when they're part of a tasty stir-fry or a side to their favorite entree, kids might not even blink an eye.

The aesthetic of food is also key. A colorful fruit salad can rival the rainbow spread of a candy display, and cleverly designed food, like smiley-faced sandwiches, can turn lunch into an adventure. We must not underestimate the power of presentation in amplifying the appeal of healthy choices.

Next, flavor is king. School lunches need to hit the flavor profiles that excite children. Spices and herbs can elevate dishes without adding unwanted sodium or sugar. A bland pea soup stands no chance, but what about a vibrant pea and mint soup, sprinkled with a touch of cheese?

It's also critical to involve children in the process. When they've had a say in choosing or even preparing their meals, there's a more significant investment in what's on their plate. This might sound like a tall order for school systems, but salad bars, build-your-own sandwich stations, and other interactive lunch line options can serve as practical solutions.

Educators and cafeteria staff can also be powerful allies in making nutritious lunches appealing. A fun fact about how astronauts eat in space can make a simple meal of chicken and rice suddenly fascinating. Or consider the influence of a lunch monitor who can't stop raving about the day's veggie chili.

Let's not forget about peer relations. Kids often want what their friends are having. Creating an environment where healthier options are the norm can catalyze a cultural shift. When the popular kid prefers a whole wheat wrap over a hot dog, others might follow suit.

While it's vital for meals to be nutritionally dense, taste can't be sacrificed. We can't serve up bowls of leafy greens and expect excitement – there has to be a hook. So, savvy meal planners might toss those greens with a scrumptious dressing or nestle them into a taco, transforming the mundane into something unexpectedly delicious.

A concern, of course, is cost. Budget constraints can make the quest for nutrition and appeal in schools feel like climbing a mountain. Yet, there are heroes in communities around the nation, innovative garden programs, and farm-to-school initiatives that are making strides. These provide fresh, appetizing produce at a fraction of the cost while also educating kids about the origin of their food.

No conversation about school lunches is complete without touching on inclusivity. We must ensure dietary restrictions and preferences are considered. Whether it's offering plant-based options or respecting religious dietary laws, we make every child feel their needs are equally important.

Ultimately, the perfect school lunch is a blend of science and soul. It combines the nutritional framework that supports a child's growth with the universal desire for joy in eating. We must weave together health facts with the threads of culture, pleasure, and community, crafting meals that sustain both the body and the spirit of our children.

Above all, we must remember, change doesn't happen overnight. There needs to be a consistent effort to adjust the lens through which children view their food. Patience, creativity, and understanding are the ingredients for revolutionizing school lunches, transforming them into meals that delight the palate while fortifying the body.

Let's seize the opportunity school lunches provide. They're a chance to make a daily impact on children's health choices, imparting lessons that can last a lifetime. As our kids line up with their trays, let it be for food that not only fuels their growth but also piques their curiosity and satisfies their zest for flavorsome meals.

In the end, it's a partnership between taste and nutrition that we're after. And when we get it right, we can watch our children's faces light up in the lunchroom – not for the flashiest packaging or the saltiest snack but for the vibrant, hearty, and utterly delightful foods that are the cornerstone of a life-long healthy relationship with eating.

Handling Birthday Parties and Sleepovers As we navigate through the various settings where our children make food choices, birthday parties and sleepovers present unique challenges. These events can often feel like obstacle courses laden with sugary temptations and treats that fall outside our carefully curated plans for a healthy diet. However, with a little preparation and savvy strategies, we can help our kids to enjoy these social occasions without completely abandoning their nutritious habits. So, let's explore how we can maintain that fine balance between festivity and well-being.

Birthday parties are often synonymous with cake, ice cream, and an array of finger foods that are more about fun than nutrition. It's important to acknowledge that a single day of indulgence won't undo healthy habits established over time. Encourage your child to enjoy the special treats on offer during birthday celebrations, but also talk to them about the idea of moderation. Simple strategies such as filling up on a healthy snack before the party or choosing smaller portions can empower your child to make smarter choices while still participating fully in the fun.

Sleepovers add another dimension to the dietary puzzle, as kids are faced with extended periods of snacking, often late into the night. Before your child heads to a sleepover, consider sending them with a healthy contribution to the snack table, such as homemade granola bars or fruit skewers. This is not only courteous to the host but also ensures that healthier options are available.

Communication is key when it comes to navigating these social events. Open a dialogue with the host parents to understand what food will be served. If your child has dietary restrictions or allergies, this step is crucial to ensure their safety. Share information about your child's needs and offer to provide suitable alternatives if necessary. Most hosts will appreciate knowing this ahead of time and will be glad to accommodate.

Role modeling plays a significant role in how children approach food choices in social settings. If they see you enjoying a wide range of foods—including occasional treats—in moderation, they're more likely to follow suit. Show enthusiasm for healthy eating, but also demonstrate that it's completely acceptable to enjoy a piece of birthday cake without guilt.

Teaching your children about balance in their diet can begin with an understanding of why we eat certain foods and the effects they have on our bodies. An educational approach can demystify the reasons behind choosing whole grains over refined sugars or reaching for water over soda. With this knowledge, children are better equipped to make conscious food choices during parties and sleepovers.

Instilling the value of listening to one's body is also beneficial. Encouraging kids to pay attention to hunger and fullness cues helps them decide when to eat and when they've had enough. This approach works at home, at school, and yes, even at birthday parties draped in streamers and dotted with balloons.

When it comes to sleepovers, breakfast is an often overlooked but important consideration. A night of less-than-ideal eating can be somewhat counterbalanced by a wholesome morning meal. Recommend to your child or discuss with the hosting parent about the possibility of having a nutrition-packed breakfast, such as oatmeal or yogurt with fresh fruit.

There's also an opportunity to use these social gatherings as a teaching moment about food-related etiquette and mindfulness. Educate your child on how to politely decline foods they don't want or that don't align with their dietary habits, as well as the importance of being grateful for what is offered.

Another method to manage the party food scene is to host your own child's events. This allows you to control the menu, providing mainly healthy options while still serving some traditional treats. Fun doesn't have to be sacrificed—create exciting themes around fruits, veggies, and other nourishing foods that appeal to the kids' sense of adventure and play.

However, the focus shouldn't always be on the food. Elevate other elements of the party or sleepover, such as games, crafts, or movie time, to ensure experiences aren't solely food-centered. These activities can occupy the kids' minds and hands, potentially lessening the emphasis on snacking.

Even with the best preparations, there will be times when your child may overindulge. Use these moments as opportunities for learning rather than sources of frustration. Talk to your child about how they feel after eating certain foods in excess and remind them of the benefits of eating a balanced diet. A tummy ache can be a memorable reminder of why we don't eat cake every day.

It's also helpful to have a conversation with your child about peer pressure and food choices. Discuss strategies for handling situations where friends may encourage eating when they're not hungry or choosing foods they usually wouldn't. Equip them with polite responses or the confidence to stick to their personal choices without feeling left out.

Finally, celebrate each small victory. Whether your child chooses water over soda, opts for fruits instead of a second serving of cake, or introduces their friends to a new, healthy snack, these are moments to be proud of. Even in party hats and pajamas, they're learning to navigate the world of nutrition, one choice at a time.

Remember, while healthy eating is a lifelong journey, it's also important to enjoy life's celebrations. By promoting balance, preparedness, and mindfulness, we can ensure that birthday parties and sleepovers contribute positively to our children's social experiences and their relationship with food.

Now, let's bake the cake and blow out the candles with confidence that we can guide our kids towards nutritional wisdom, even in a room filled with balloons and laughter. Next, we'll continue on to examine how cooking and baking are not only fun activities but also invaluable educational tools that cement healthy eating practices.

Chapter 12:
Cooking and Baking as Learning Tools

Stepping into the kitchen, children embark on a culinary adventure that transcends the mere act of meal preparation. Cooking and baking can transform into incredible learning spheres, where measuring cups and spices bring math and science to life. Imagine the look of amazement on your child's face as they watch yeast spring to life in a warm bowl, or learn fractions while dividing a pizza—these are the moments that demystify abstract concepts with delectable clarity. The act of stirring, pouring, and tasting isn't just about the creation of a dish; it's a hands-on education on nutrition and the vital role each ingredient plays in our bodies. Sifting through the myriad of colors, textures, and flavors, children develop a palatable vocabulary that fosters an appreciation of wholesome, nutrient-filled foods. Every whisk and knead strengthens not only fine motor skills but also the bond between caregiver and child, cementing healthy habits and heartwarming memories. So, let's turn our kitchens into classrooms where patience is practiced, creativity flourishes, and a little bit of mess is just part of the delicious discovery.

Engaging Kids in the Kitchen Cooking can be a carnival of colors, flavors, and textures—an experience that's both educational and enjoyable. It's a fantastic place for learning and a playground for bonding. When kids get involved in the kitchen, they're not just learning how to cook, they're gaining valuable skills and developing a deeper relationship with food. Let's explore ways to make the kitchen inviting, fun, and an informative space for little chefs-to-be.

First and foremost, safety is key. Children need to understand the importance of washing hands, keeping work surfaces clean, and respecting kitchen tools, especially anything sharp or hot. Explain these practices with patience and care before starting any culinary activity. Safety guidelines will become second nature through consistent reinforcement, leaving more room for the fun stuff.

Start small. For the youngest in the fold, even toddlers can wash fruits and veggies or mix salad with their clean little hands. Keep it simple and let them feel a sense of accomplishment with these basic tasks. Gradually, as their confidence and curiosity grow, so can their responsibilities. Give them a chance to measure, pour, and stir, always under watchful but not overbearing eyes.

Interactive experiences work wonders with children. Plan a 'make your own pizza' night or a 'build-a-bowl' event where kids can choose from a variety of healthy toppings. Through this, they're learning about food groups and nutrition without even realizing it. It's a perfect segue into talking about where foods come from, their benefits, and why a colorful plate means a wealth of nutrients.

When it comes to older kids, assigning them a 'special project' like preparing a family dinner once a week can be ideal. It teaches them planning, time management, and the joy of seeing others savor the meals they've prepared. Guidance is crucial but resist the urge to take over. Be a cheerleader by their side, not the coach that calls every play.

Think about investing in kid-friendly kitchen tools. A set of knives suited for smaller hands, lightweight mixing bowls, and colorful measuring cups can make the experience more accessible and appealing. These tools help kids feel like the kitchen is a place for them, too—not just the grown-ups.

For many children, baking is a natural entry point into the world of cooking. The precision required for baking is a teachable moment for following directions and the magic of science—the way ingredients transform with heat or mix together to create something delicious generates excitement and interest.

To keep the momentum going, get kids involved in the meal planning process. Let them pick a recipe or two for the week. By giving them a voice in what comes to the table, they're more invested in the outcome—a powerful motivator to get involved and try new foods.

Mistakes will happen, and that's perfectly fine. A pancake that turns out too crispy or a salad slightly overdressed can be learning experiences. Encourage children to taste and tweak, discussing what might improve the dish next time. This critical thinking develops palate education and builds resilience—not every experiment will be perfect, but every attempt is valuable.

Take advantage of seasonal foods and festivities. Carving pumpkins, picking apples, and shelling peas can all be precursors to cooking. When kids are involved in the full process—from field to plate—they develop a deep appreciation for the food they eat.

Don't forget to talk about portions and balance while cooking. As you add ingredients, discuss their roles in the meal—are they adding protein, fiber, or vitamins? How much is enough? This conversation can flow naturally and is more tangible when there's visual and hands-on learning.

In the bustle of cooking, patience can sometimes wear thin. Remember to breathe and embrace the mess. A kitchen splattered with some flour and laughter is a sign of a family growing together. It's easier to wipe up spills than it is to undo a negative experience that can push kids away from wanting to participate.

Display the fruits of labor—when a meal or snack is ready, present it proudly. Celebrate the effort put into the creation. A simple "You made this!" can ignite a beaming smile and a sense of pride. This positive reinforcement fuels the desire to cook and learn more.

Incorporate feedback sessions post-meal where you can discuss what everyone thought about the food. Children feel respected when their opinions are solicited and valued. Keep the conversation constructive and uplifting.

Lastly, remember to be present. It's not just about the delicious food but the memories made along the way. The ultimate goal is to build a love for healthy eating and cooking that they will carry with them into adulthood—one diced carrot and teaspoon at a time.

Fostering a child's interest in the kitchen is a gift that keeps on giving. It nurtures independence, awareness of nutrition, and family connections. It's a blend of education and entertainment that can shape a child's approach to food for a lifetime. Engaging them early sets the stage for a future where they're able to make healthier choices, appreciate the diversity of foods, and enjoy the act of cooking as a fundamental, yet joyful part of daily life.

Teaching Nutrition Through Cooking Activities employs the engaging and hands-on experience of food preparation to instill fundamental nutritional concepts in kids. Engaging young minds in this practical process turns abstract ideas about healthy eating into tangible, memorable events. By approaching cooking with energy and creativity, these activities can transform the way children view nutrition entirely.

Let's face it—children are playful and naturally curious beings, eager to touch, taste, and experiment. Cooking offers the perfect realm for this exploration. Imagine a child's wonder as they roll dough for the first time or pick herbs from a garden to flavor a dish—it's sensory learning at its best. In these magical kitchen moments, we have an unparalleled opportunity to talk about where food comes from, its nutritional value, and how it helps our bodies thrive.

Initiating this educational foray doesn't require elaborate equipment or a professional culinary background. Start small—mixing a salad or assembling a fruit parfait—and emphasize the colors, textures, and flavors involved. Describe how the bright reds of strawberries or the deep greens of spinach are not just visually pleasing but packed with vitamins that power their play.

Advance through more complex tasks as children grow in confidence and skill. Measuring ingredients for a stir-fry introduces math and science concepts while opening discussions about the vitamins in peppers or the fiber in brown rice. Bake some bread, and let the yeast's magic spark a conversation on chemical reactions, and then segue into the benefits of whole grains over refined flours.

Keep in mind the importance of inclusivity in these activities. Invite children to share family recipes or dishes significant to their culture. This won't just expand their palates but also instill a respect for nutritional diversity and the stories that food tells about us.

Understandably, safety is paramount. Always supervise closely and steer young chefs toward age-appropriate tasks. The goal here is to build their skills and knowledge without risking injury. In doing so, we not only teach about nutrition but also imbue them with a sense of responsibility and safety consciousness.

Now, let's talk about balance—the cornerstone of a nutritious diet. Cooking activities provide an environment to learn how to balance the plate with protein, whole grains, fruits, veggies, and healthy fats. For instance, assembling their own tacos can teach children to moderate high-calorie toppings and focus on fresh, nutrient-packed ingredients.

Portion control is another vital lesson easily integrated into cooking. Explain why piling a plate too high might lead to overeating, and let them serve themselves to practice moderation. Use visual cues like the size of their fist to estimate appropriate serving sizes, making the concept relatable and easier to grasp.

Don't underestimate the power of themed cooking projects. A 'rainbow day', where each dish includes fruits and veggies of a different color, visually reinforces the idea of eating a variety of foods to get all the essential nutrients. It's fun, it's memorable, and it's effective.

Interlink cooking with the food choices they make outside of home. Prepare a common fast food meal together using wholesome ingredients and compare it with the store-bought version. These activities cultivate critical thinking about the foods they choose and encourage them to prioritize homemade meals.

Sustainability is a critical topic that can be woven into cooking lessons. Use ingredients from a local farmers' market or start a mini herb garden to explain the environmental benefits of local and homegrown produce. Kids are the leaders of tomorrow, and eco-conscious eating habits can start today.

Timing is everything. Introduce these activities when children are most receptive, such as after school or on the weekend when there's less rush. The patience you display and the joy you express as you cook together will stick with them more than any nutritional fact.

Remember, the end product doesn't have to be perfect. If the soup is a bit salty or the cake slightly sunken, it's okay. The focus should be on the experience and the nutritional knowledge gained, not just on the output. Celebrate the effort and the willingness to try new things, and they'll be more likely to continue cooking and experimenting with healthy foods in the future.

Finally, reinforce the lessons. Talk about the day's cooking at dinner or reference it when grocery shopping together. Embedding nutrition education in multiple facets of life consolidates those insights and makes healthy eating a natural, instinctive part of growing up.

Cooking activities are not just about teaching nutrition; they're about sharing moments, passing on values, and cooking up a lifetime's worth of healthy habits. So let's roll up our sleeves, warm up the oven, and get ready to change lives, one recipe at a time.

Chapter 13:
Cultural Considerations in Child Nutrition

Imagine the colorful tapestry of world cultures, each strand woven with its own unique flavors, textures, and nutritional philosophies. In Chapter 13, we dive into the rich mosaic of cultural considerations that play a pivotal role in child nutrition. Here, we'll unpack the importance of acknowledging and respecting diverse dietary traditions while guiding children towards a nutritionally balanced diet. It's about celebrating the kaleidoscope of edible heritages and integrating these vibrant foodways into children's meals in a way that nurtures both body and spirit. By nurturing an understanding and appreciation for the wide array of cultural cuisines, we empower kids to explore a global palate with excitement and open-mindedness. Equipping them with this culinary curiosity not only helps broaden their tastes but also instills a profound respect for the varied ways people around the world sustain and delight themselves. This chapter isn't just about what's on the plate; it's about how the stories, traditions, and values behind those foods can enrich our children's lives and palates.

Respecting Diverse Dietary Traditions As we navigate the landscape of child nutrition, it's paramount to acknowledge and honor the rich tapestry of cultural diversity that shapes dietary traditions. Families across the globe follow an array of eating practices rooted in history, tradition, and belief, making the 'one size fits all' approach to nutrition education impractical, if not impossible. This section sheds light on how we can respect, understand, and incorporate these diverse dietary traditions when guiding children towards healthy eating habits.

First and foremost, let's recognize that food is much more than mere nourishment; it's a vibrant language through which cultures express their identity. Meals crafted in households are often recipes passed down through generations, imbued with tales and traditions. Acknowledging these traditions is fundamental in fostering a well-rounded eating habit in children that does not alienate their cultural heritage but rather celebrates it.

That said, balancing cultural dishes with nutritional needs can be a delicate dance. It's not about discarding traditional foods but about finding ways to tweak and incorporate them into a balanced diet. This often involves playing with portion sizes, preparation methods, and ingredient choices to enhance nutritional value while keeping cultural significance intact.

Education is key here. It's important to engage children in discussions about various dietary customs and why some families may prefer certain foods over others—be it for health, religious reasons, economic factors, or sustainability. These conversations can broaden children's perspectives and foster inclusivity and respect among peers with different dietary traditions.

In today's global village, exposure to a world of cuisines is at our fingertips. Encouraging trying new foods from different cultures can be an exhilarating educational venture for kids. Making this an adventure rather than a chore enhances their appreciation for diversity and broadens their palate—and it's fun, too!

When addressing the subject of diverse dietary traditions in educational settings, sensitivity and inclusivity are non-negotiable. Caregivers and educators should be well-informed and cautious so as not to stereotype or make assumptions about certain cultural practices.

Approaching these topics with curiosity and respect sets the tone for the children's own attitudes.

Let's also consider religious observances that impact food choices, such as kosher, halal, or vegetarian diets. Teaching children the reasons behind these diets not only deepens their own understanding but also builds empathy for peers who may have strict dietary guidelines based on their religious beliefs.

Meal planning presents a unique opportunity to fuse traditional recipes with contemporary nutritional needs. By involving children in selecting recipes from their own—or a classmate's—cultural background, they learn about the ingredients and their nutritional benefits. This approach transforms meal preparation into a multicultural event that nourishes both body and mind.

Moreover, respecting dietary traditions means being aware of the socio-economic factors that influence food availability. We must consider these constraints when recommending changes or adaptations to a family's dietary habits, thereby avoiding any unintentional cultural insensitivity or imposition of dominant food narratives.

It is crucial to forge partnerships with parents and caregivers from diverse backgrounds, creating open channels of communication wherein they feel comfortable sharing their cultural practices. This way, educators and healthcare professionals can customize nutrition education to be culturally responsive and relevant.

Take for instance the importance of community events, like potlucks or food fairs, where children can experience an array of dishes from various cultures. These events aren't just about food; they're celebratory learning experiences that validate and esteem diverse dietary traditions.

Within this context, we must also address language barriers that may impede a shared understanding of nutrition. Offering educational materials in multiple languages and employing interpreters when necessary can significantly improve the effectiveness of nutrition education programs in diverse communities.

Another critical topic is the misrepresentation or misunderstanding of cultural foods in media and how it influences children's perceptions. It's our job to counteract potential stereotypes by portraying traditional diets in an accurate and positive light with the same respect given to popular Western diets.

Lastly, while the focus here has been on respecting diverse dietary traditions, it's equally important to highlight the common ground all cultures share: the universal importance of nutritious foods for growth and development. Emphasizing this shared goal unites us all in the endeavor to raise healthy kids.

By embracing diversity in dietary traditions, we enrich children's lives through food. It's through this multifaceted lens that we can truly appreciate the complexity and beauty of feeding our next generation. It's not just about food; it's teaching children about respect, open-mindedness, and the acceptance of differences, setting the foundation for a healthier, more unified world.

Incorporating Cultural Foods into a Balanced Diet When it comes to nourishing our children, it's essential to remember that healthy eating doesn't mean forgoing the rich tapestry of cultural foods that many families hold dear. In fact, embracing these foods can be a fantastic way to foster a balanced and nutritious diet while celebrating heritage and diversity. Every culture has its staples, its comfort food, and those special dishes reserved for festive occasions. It's about finding a harmony between traditional culinary customs and the principles of modern nutrition.

Now, imagine the vibrancy of a plate filled with the colorful vegetables found in traditional Caribbean dishes or the variety of spices that lace the fragrant curries of South Asia. These are not just flavorsome experiences; they're opportunities to introduce children to a world of nutrients. Foods like legumes, grains, nuts, fruits, and vegetables are central in many cultural diets and are also powerhouses of essential vitamins and minerals.

Let's talk about balance. Integrating cultural foods into a child's diet means considering the roles and proportions of macronutrients—carbohydrates, proteins, and fats—as well as vitamins and minerals. Take, for instance, the Mediterranean diet, which is lauded for its balanced approach, weaving together grains, fish, olive oil, and a medley of plant foods that are as nourishing as they are delicious. This dietary pattern encapsulates a balance that many cultures can emulate and modify as per their culinary traditions.

It's also about flexibility and creativity. Often, traditional dishes can be adapted to boost their nutritional profile. Substituting refined grains with their whole counterparts, opting for healthier fats, or incorporating a greater variety of fruits and vegetables can enhance the health benefits of cultural recipes without sacrificing taste or significance.

Portion control is another vital aspect of incorporating cultural foods. While certain dishes might be rich in healthy ingredients, their caloric content should still be factored into the day's overall intake. Offering children smaller portions of rich foods alongside larger servings of vegetables and fruits can maintain nutritional balance.

In some instances, traditional dishes might be centered around meat or dairy, which can be high in saturated fats. One way to navigate this is to integrate these items into meals in a way that respects their cultural importance while still moderating intake. For instance, using meat as a garnish or flavor enhancer rather than the main component of a dish can make a substantial difference.

Fostering an appreciation for cultural foods also means teaching children about the significance behind what they're eating. Sharing stories of the origins of dishes, the traditional ways they're prepared, and the celebrations they're associated with, helps build a deeper respect and understanding of their own and others' cultures.

Encouraging children to explore a variety of cultural foods can be a sensory adventure that expands their palate while providing a spectrum of nutrients. For instance, exposing them to Japanese cuisine can introduce them to seaweed, a great source of iodine, or teaching them about the use of pulses in Indian cooking can highlight great sources of plant-based protein.

In multicultural societies, children often have peers from different backgrounds, making shared meals an excellent opportunity for cultural exchange. Potlucks, community events, and even school lunches can provide windows into other cultures and serve as educational moments about balanced eating within different dietary traditions.

Combining cultural foods with the fundamentals of nutrition requires a curious mind and willingness to experiment. There's joy in discovering new foods and reinventing recipes to boost their healthfulness. Encouraging kids to partake in this process not only educates them but also sparks a sense of excitement and ownership over what they eat.

Let's also consider the role of spices and herbs, which are staples in many cultural cuisines. Aside from adding depth and complexity to dishes, many have health-promoting properties. Turmeric, ginger, garlic, and cinnamon are just a few examples with notable benefits. They can turn a simple meal into a symphony of flavor and nutrition.

Moreover, teaching kids about the traditional ways foods are prepared and consumed can offer important nutritional lessons. For instance, fermentation—a process widely used in Korean, European, and African cuisines—not only preserves food but also creates probiotics that are beneficial for gut health.

Remember, agonizing over the "perfect" diet can be counterproductive, especially when it risks overlooking the pleasures of shared cultural experiences. It's about crafting a narrative of nutrition that's inclusive, not exclusive, one that celebrates diversity and promotes health simultaneously. The goal isn't to remove cultural foods from the equation but rather to integrate them intelligently and with joy.

Ultimately, incorporating cultural foods into a balanced diet is an ongoing journey, not a one-time goal. It's an evolving practice where recipes are handed down, adapted, and perhaps even improved with nutrition in mind. It's about drawing from the past to enrich the present and future health of our children.

Weaving cultural foods into a balanced diet can be a foundation for life-long healthy eating habits. It's a chance to educate, appreciate, and savor the multitude of flavors our world offers. And most importantly, it's a way to pass on a legacy of health and heritage to the young minds we nurture.

Chapter 14:
Technology and Nutritional Education

In an era where screen time is as much a part of our daily routine as meal times, it's pivotal to harness the power of technology in laying the groundwork for smart nutritional choices in children. By turning our attention to interactive apps and engaging digital resources, we've got the world at our fingertips to make nutritional education not just informative but downright fun. Think of it: vibrant apps that transform calorie counting into a game, social platforms where parents and kids cheer on each other's healthy choices, or virtual communities that serve as a touchstone for support and awareness. These digital wonders aren't just about swiping and clicking; they're potential goldmines for fostering a culture of well-informed, food-savvy kids. From tracking the rainbow of fruits and veggies they consume, to understanding the nitty-gritty of what makes a balanced meal, technology invites a level of interaction and personalization that traditional methods can't match, bridging the gap between learning and doing. So let's leverage these tools to create an engaging, supportive environment where children learn to make well-rounded nutritional choices that'll stick with them for life.

Using Apps and Digital Resources to nurture a healthy relationship with food can feel like a balancing act. But, let's dive into the digital age where a plethora of tools awaits to make this journey fun and educational. It's not uncommon to worry about screen time, yet, in controlled doses, technology can be a wonderful ally in teaching kids about nutrition and helping them track their eating habits.

We're witnessing an exciting era where a smartphone or tablet can become a learning hub for children. A carefully selected app might hold the power to transform a mundane task into an interactive game, where children earn rewards and a sense of accomplishment, all while learning to make healthier food choices. Imagine an app that turns choosing veggies into a heroic quest, or a food diary that rewards children with fun animations for adding fruits to their daily intake—yes, those exist!

Let's zero in on digital tools that educate. Many apps have been developed with young users in mind, featuring colorful graphics and engaging content that covertly delivers powerful lessons about nutrition. They toe the line between entertainment and education, often referred to as 'edutainment', ensuring that children remain engrossed as they absorb valuable information.

Digital resources also offer a unique way to track nutritional intake. For older kids and teens, tracking apps can be both eye-opening and empowering. They learn to be mindful of what they eat and make connections between their food choices and how they feel. It's about making data approachable and actionable for improving their diets.

Moreover, alongside apps, there are interactive websites. These platforms can offer a depth and breadth of information in a way that's engaging for children. With recipes, videos, quizzes, and even virtual tours of farms or factories, these websites can unveil the journey food takes from farm to plate, fostering a greater understanding and appreciation for what ends up on their dinner table.

However, it's critical to navigate this space with a sense of discernment. Not all health and nutrition apps are created equal, and some might even carry misleading information. Hence, it's key to choose those endorsed by healthcare or nutritional professionals and avoid apps that promote calorie counting, which can encourage an unhealthy focus on numbers rather than overall well-being.

Educational videos also open up a world of possibilities for learning. They can bring concepts to life that might otherwise be abstract in a child's mind. Explainer videos about the digestive system or the role of different nutrients create a visual narrative that children can relate to and understand.

Then there's the social aspect. Many digital tools provide a platform for children to connect with peers who have similar dietary goals or challenges, such as food allergies. In this safe digital space, they can share stories, swap recipes, and support one another. It's about forming a community that encourages positive food choices and a collective learning experience.

The right app can also be a boon for parents and caregivers. With features that help plan balanced meals, generate shopping lists, and provide nutritional tips, these apps can take the stress out of meal prep and ensure that children are getting the right nutrition. Think less guesswork and more efficient grocery trips.

And what about fitness trackers? Most people associate them with adults hitting the gym, but they can also be adapted for children. They can monitor physical activity levels and encourage children to move more, which is fundamentally interlinked with their nutritional health.

In today's fast-paced world, convenience matters. Digital cookbooks and online meal planning services can introduce fresh, healthy recipes that cater to a child's palate and dietary needs. With step-by-step instructions and detailed nutritional information at your fingertips, preparing wholesome meals can become less daunting and more achievable.

One must also address the reality of "gamification" in the context of nutrition. Gamified apps that include challenges, levels, and rewards can motivate children by giving them tangible goals to reach in their nutritional journeys. This approach turns the education process into a game where each healthy choice takes them a step further.

Digital books and e-readers deserve a mention too. They provide access to a myriad of cookbooks, nutritional guides, and food stories suitable for a range of age groups. It's about giving children a library of resources that they can dig into any time they're curious—it's empowerment through information at their own pace.

Lastly, let's not forget podcasts and audiobooks. For auditory learners, these can be a goldmine. Listening to family-friendly podcasts about healthy eating or stories that revolve around healthy food adventures can influence children's perspectives on nutrition without them ever having to look at a screen.

Ultimately, apps and digital resources are tools—and like all tools, their effectiveness hinges on how they are used. Integrating them thoughtfully into a child's life can change the narrative of nutrition education, making it a dynamic and interactive process. Harnessing the power of these tools can help pave the way towards a future of informed, health-conscious individuals embarking on their lifelong journey of healthy eating.

The Role of Virtual Communities in Support and Awareness
In our hyper-connected world, virtual communities have become a vibrant lifeline for parents and caregivers aiming to foster healthier eating habits in children. The term 'virtual communities' refers to groups of people who interact, exchange ideas, and support each other through the internet. For individuals seeking encouragement or guidance on child nutrition, these online ecosystems can be as crucial as a well-stocked pantry.

Imagine this scene: it's late at night, the house is quiet, but a parent's mind is buzzing with concerns about their child's eating behavior. Where does one turn? Online forums, social media groups, and specialized support communities are now just a few clicks away. Here, people exchange stories, swap recipes, and find a sense of togetherness in the journey for better health.

This digital camaraderie fosters awareness far beyond the capabilities of individual research. Parents discover not only what to serve at the dinner table but also how to handle the emotional and psychological aspects of feeding children. These tidbits of shared wisdom can lead to more than just mealtime victories—they support the development of long-lasting, healthy eating behaviors.

Within these virtual havens, members celebrate each other's successes. When a child who's been a picky eater tries a new vegetable, it's championed. Or when a parent finds a way to incorporate more whole foods into snacks, it's applauded. Shared success stories are potent motivators, and the ripple effect of a single victory can be extensive and profound.

Furthermore, online communities offer a stage for various experts—nutritionists, pediatricians, and dietitians—to provide professional insights. Through webinars, Q&A sessions, or informative posts, child nutrition is demystified, empowering parents to make informed decisions for the well-being of their families.

These platforms also amplify the significance of awareness, dedication, and the proactive pursuit of knowledge. Being part of a virtual community equips caregivers with the tools needed not just to react to challenges, but to anticipate them. Say 'goodbye' to being blindsided by the latest snack trend, and 'hello' to having preemptive strategies for balancing treats with nutritious offerings.

One might assume that the impersonal nature of the internet could reduce the meaningfulness of these interactions. However, the opposite is often true—digital connections can provide a level of anonymity that fosters open, honest exchanges that might be harder to come by in face-to-face settings.

These communities also serve as a feedback loop for raising awareness on the latest research in child nutrition. Discussions on groundbreaking studies quickly disseminate through these networks, prompting parents to adapt new evidence-based practices into their routines.

Moreover, virtual communities serve as a sounding board for parents to voice their concerns and challenges. When it feels like nobody in one's immediate circle understands the struggles of managing a child's food allergies or dealing with a fussy eater, this online family steps up with both empathy and practical advice.

But it's not just about having a place to vent or seek comfort— these virtual spaces can become a robust hub for initiating change in the broader community. Advocacy start-ups, crowd-funding for food education programs, and campaigns for healthier school lunches have all found kindling in the engine room of online forums.

Accessibility is yet another hallmark of these digital clusters. No matter where one lives—be it a buzzing city or a remote rural area—the internet has dissolved geographical barriers. Support and understanding are no longer constrained by one's locale, ensuring that every parent has the chance to be heard and to learn.

The knowledge shared within these groups extends to handling difficult social scenarios, too. From navigating the complex dynamics at family dinners to making intelligent choices at the cafeteria, virtual communities provide strategic wisdom that underpin these real-world situations.

At the heart of these communities lies a collective wisdom that transcends individual experience. The collective is always learning, always teaching—a living repository of shared experiences that affirms the notion that in unity there is strength.

These online support systems can also act as a compass for parents floundering in the sea of misinformation that often floods the internet. They help debunk myths and underline the importance of seeking credible, scientifically-backed advice on child nutrition.

In closing, the role of virtual communities in support and awareness for healthy child nutrition is as diverse as it is substantial. They provide a tapestry of resources where one can draw inspiration, find solace, and gather the strength to implement positive changes, all within arm's reach of a keyboard or touchscreen. For parents and caregivers navigating the nuanced world of child nutrition, these virtual communities are not just beneficial—they're indispensable.

Conclusion

As we come to the close of our collective journey through the essential world of child nutrition, it's time to take a moment to reflect on the wisdom we've gathered and the tools we now possess to nurture the health and wellbeing of our children. The knowledge we've covered, spanning from the foundational aspects of nutrition to coping with dietary challenges and leveraging technology, serves as our guide in an often complex food landscape.

We've explored the building blocks of nutrition and the pivotal role that macronutrients and micronutrients play in the growth and development of our young ones. Understanding this is not just academic; it empowers us to make choices that fortify our children's bodies and foster their potential.

Establishing healthy eating habits early on is akin to planting seeds in a well-tended garden. We learned the value of creating positive food environments and the transformative power of routine. By nurturing these habits, we lay the groundwork for a lifetime of well-being.

As busy parents and caregivers, we often find meal planning to be daunting, but we've discussed strategies to make it approachable and enjoyable. The concept of the Mighty Kids' Plate is a testament to the idea that balanced and enticing meals can be both nutritious and satisfying.

Facing the challenges of picky eaters or fast-paced lifestyles has led us to innovate in our approaches to diet. We're reminded of the influence that we, as parents, hold over our children's food choices. By modeling healthy behaviors, we serve as live-in mentors for how to engage with food mindfully.

The bond between diet and physical activity has become clear as we discovered the critical nature of movement in our children's lives. Like a symphony, exercise, and nutrition play together to support robust growth and boundless energy.

In considering the impact of food choices on our planet, we took steps toward sustainable eating practices. It's not just about the now; it's about setting a stage for a healthy planet where our children can thrive in the future.

Addressing food allergies and dietary restrictions reminded us of the importance of vigilance and education. We are armed with the know-how to navigate the sometimes tricky terrain of keeping our kids safe and well-nurtured despite these challenges.

When it comes to snacks, we now see the opportunity to choose whole foods over processed options and inspire our children with creative and healthy selections. The insights shared on hydration further our commitment to prioritizing water intake over sugary alternatives.

The social aspect of eating, especially in school settings and during recreational gatherings, presents its own set of navigational cues. We've grasped methods for managing nutritional quality without compromising the joy of social meals and events.

Bringing our kids into the kitchen provides an exceptional learning environment. Through cooking and baking activities, we're teaching them practical skills and nutritional knowledge in one of the most hands-on methods possible.

We acknowledged the beautiful diversity of dietary traditions, respecting and integrating them into the rich tapestry of a balanced dietary lifestyle. By doing so, we celebrate our heritage and the broad range of nutritious foods available to us.

Technology has proven itself an ally in the quest for nutritional education, offering apps and virtual communities that stand as testament to innovation in support and awareness. With these digital resources, we stay connected and informed, no matter where our busy lives might lead us.

Finally, as we equip ourselves with the array of healthy, nutrient-rich recipes and tools compiled in the appendices, we do so with a sense of capability and optimism. Our role as educators, parents, and caregivers is clear: to be the guiding light that leads our children toward habits that will sustain a lifetime of health and happiness.

In closing, remember that the journey does not end here. With every meal, snack, and beverage, we weave the fabric of our children's health. Let us take the knowledge we have gained and put it into daily practice. Together, we have the power to shape a future where every child is empowered to make choices that not only nourish their bodies but also nurture their spirits and minds.

Appendix A:
Appendix

As we bring our exploration of nurturing healthy eating habits in children to a close, it's key to remember that knowledge is most valuable when it's applied. In this appendix, we're not simply summarizing what we've learned; we're extending a hand to help you step confidently into action. Here you'll find a curated selection of resources that can bring the previous chapters to life in your own kitchen and daily routine, empowering you and the children in your care to embark on a journey towards sustainable health and joyous living.

Nutrient-rich Recipes for Mighty Kids

Getting kids to love wholesome food starts with the fun of cooking and the joy of shared meals. We've put together a collection of delightful recipes packed with the nutrition they need and the flavors they'll love. From smoothies laden with hidden greens to scrumptious snacks that outdo any processed temptation, these recipes are sure to inspire your little ones to explore the world of healthy tastes.

Superhero Spinach Pancakes - A vibrant way to start the day, these pancakes are as fun to look at as they are to eat.

Broccoli and Cheese Mini Muffins - Perfect for packing in lunch boxes or for a grab-and-go snack, these muffins pack both protein and veggies.

Fiesta Bean Salad - Infuse some excitement into your routine with this colorful, fiber-rich dish.

Helpful Resources and Tools

Navigating the wealth of information - and misinformation - about nutrition can be daunting. We've compiled a selection of credible resources to expand your knowledge and provide practical guidance. From printable portion guides to interactive meal planners, these tools can make healthy eating simpler and more enjoyable for everyone involved.

Centers for Disease Control and Prevention (CDC) - check out their "Kids' Quest" on nutrition for interactive learning.

USDA's ChooseMyPlate - offering meal planning guidance and educational resources tailored for different age groups.

American Academy of Pediatrics - a treasure trove of parenting tips pertaining to nutrition and health.

As you dive into these recipes and resources, remember that you're setting the stage for lifelong health and happiness. With every nutritious meal you prepare and every smart choice you make, you're not only fueling young bodies but also nurturing young minds to appreciate the power that lies in thoughtful, balanced eating. Let's raise a generation that thrives on good food and even better health.

Nutrient-rich Recipes for Mighty Kids As we continue on our journey to nourish the young ones in our care, let's roll up our sleeves and dive into a treasure trove of nutrient-rich recipes tailored for growing bodies and minds. Creating meals that appeal to kids while packing in the essential vitamins, minerals, and macronutrients can be a delightful challenge. Let's meet it head-on with enthusiasm and creativity.

Fueling our children with dietary superstars means thinking outside the box of conventional kids' menus. It's about integrating whole grains, lean proteins, healthy fats, and an abundance of fruits and vegetables in ways that tantalize young taste buds. Remember, every meal is an opportunity to build a stronger, healthier future for our kids.

Picture the breakfast table set with a smoothie bowl bursting with colorful fruits, chia seeds, and a swirl of nut butter. It's a visual feast that invites kids to dive in, and every spoonful supports their bodies with fiber, antioxidants, and essential fats. Breakfast like these set the tone for a day filled with energy and focus, essential for young scholars and adventurers alike.

Moving on to lunch, imagine a rainbow wrap, each color representing a different nutrient. From leafy greens and bright bell peppers to purple cabbage and sweet corn, these wraps are fun for kids to eat and are bursting with vitamins and fiber. Add in some lean turkey or chickpeas, and you've got a protein-packed meal that will sustain them through their afternoon activities.

The almighty after-school snack doesn't have to be a nutritional afterthought. Instead of reaching for pre-packaged options, why not offer apple "nachos"? Thinly sliced apples drizzled with a little bit of melted dark chocolate and a sprinkle of crushed nuts make for a playful and antioxidant-rich treat that kids will love assembling themselves.

For dinner, let's spin the globe and take inspiration from around the world. A hearty black bean and sweet potato stew, inspired by Latin American flavors, not only warms the belly but also supplies a hefty dose of iron, fiber, and complex carbohydrates. It's a velvety concoction that invites children to explore new tastes while nourishing their bodies.

And who says pizza can't be nutritious? Swap out the thick, greasy crust for a thin whole-grain base and top it with an array of veggies, a modest sprinkling of cheese, and a protein like shredded chicken or diced tofu. Suddenly, pizza night is transformed into an engaging way for kids to 'eat their veggies' without a fuss.

Your mighty kids will also adore interactive meals, like build-your-own taco stations. Load up the table with options like grilled fish, black beans, avocado slices, and an array of chopped veggies. This not only empowers kids to make their own choices but also gets them excited about combining flavors and nutrients in their custom creations.

Let's not forget the power of a well-crafted side dish. Something as simple as roasted carrots, seasoned with a whisper of honey and a sprinkle of thyme, can become a favorite. It's a sweet and savory way to introduce more beta-carotene into their diet, important for vision and immune health.

Desserts can certainly find a place in a nutrient-rich diet, especially when they're thoughtfully prepared. Baked pears with a dollop of yogurt and a sprinkle of cinnamon can satisfy a sweet tooth, all the while providing a boost of fiber and calcium.

When dealing with picky eaters, hidden-veggie recipes can be your best friend. Think smooth, creamy sauces for pasta made from pureed veggies, or muffins dotted with zucchini and banana for moisture and a punch of nutrients. Kids love them, and you'll love knowing they're getting an extra serving of veggies.

Involving the kids in the process of meal preparation can make them more invested in the food they eat. Try having them help mix a salad or arrange fruit on a platter. It's a subtle way to teach them about nutrition and the appeal of whole foods.

For those busy weeknights when time is scarce, fear not. Quick, nutritious meals like stir-fried brown rice with vegetables and shredded rotisserie chicken can come to the rescue. It's fast, it's easy, and it's balanced—laying the groundwork for a lifetime of healthy, stress-free dinners.

Finally, the triumph of a nutrient-rich family meal can be a fusion dish that brings together the best of all worlds — a quinoa bowl topped with a medley of stir-fried veggies, avocado, and a drizzle of a flavorful tahini-lemon dressing. It's packed with protein, healthy fats, and a wide spectrum of micronutrients, making it a power bowl fit for the mightiest of kids.

These recipes are more than just fuel; they embody the love, care, and hope we have for our young ones. By offering nutrient-rich foods, presented in a way that's fun and appealing, we're setting the stage for robust health, vibrant growth, and a lifelong appreciation for the bounty that nature provides. The recipes we've explored together are stepping stones toward that goal — delicious, nutritious, and just right for your mighty kids.

Helpful Resources and Tools As we've explored various aspects of promoting healthy eating habits in children, it's time to arm ourselves with an array of resources and tools that can make this journey smoother and more effective. Whether you're a parent, educator, or healthcare professional, having a toolkit at your disposal is invaluable. These resources can offer guidance, support, and concrete strategies to encourage kids on their path to nutritional well-being.

First and foremost, an essential component of any nutritional toolkit is reliable information sources. The United States Department of Agriculture (USDA) provides a wealth of knowledge through its website, including the MyPlate initiative, which has replaced the traditional food pyramid. MyPlate is a fantastic visual guide that illustrates the portions and variety of foods that should be included in a balanced meal, tailored specifically for kids.

Another gem is the American Academy of Pediatrics (AAP). Their website and publications delve deep into the nuances of child nutrition, from breastfeeding and weaning to managing nutrition for athletes in their teenage years. They also address diverse topics such as eating disorders and obesity prevention, catering to a broad spectrum of needs and concerns.

Don't underestimate the power of a good cookbook – especially one designed with kids in mind. Cookbooks targeted at preparing meals for children can inspire creativity, introduce new foods, and help you plan balanced meals with recipes that have been dietitian-approved.

Technology also plays a significant role in today's world, and there are several reputable apps and websites that offer meal planning, grocery shopping, and nutrition tracking specifically tailored for children. Look for those that have engaging interfaces for the kids and came from credible sources, ensuring they foster healthy eating without promoting unnecessary restrictions.

Interactive games and activities can be exceptionally effective in teaching children about nutrition. Online platforms and even certain board games turn learning about food groups, vitamins, and minerals into fun experiences that can help solidify these concepts in young minds.

Beyond digital resources, it's essential to have tangible tools within your home or classroom. Measuring cups, food models, and portion plates can make abstract ideas about portions and food groups much clearer for children. There's real magic when kids can get their hands on these tools and explore for themselves.

Gardening kits or projects might sound unconventional when talking about nutrition, but they can be a fantastic resource. Being involved in growing their fruits and vegetables can encourage children to try and enjoy a broader range of fresh produce, building a connection between the earth and their eating habits.

Support groups and workshops for parents and caregivers can also be helpful, providing a space to share experiences, challenges, and strategies. Often, local health departments, libraries, or community centers offer classes or meetings where you can connect with others who are focusing on child nutrition.

For those managing food allergies or intolerances, it can feel overwhelming trying to navigate dietary restrictions. Organizations such as Food Allergy Research & Education (FARE) offer comprehensive guidelines, alternative recipes, and educational materials to keep your child both safe and well-nourished.

Label reading is an essential skill for ensuring your child is eating healthy foods, and there are quick-reference guides and charts available that can help streamline this process. These can help you and your child understand what's truly in the foods you are considering and make better-informed decisions.

Remember the aspect of physical activity discussed in earlier chapters? Be sure to have a list of community sports teams, activity clubs, and other resources that promote active play. This ties into nutritional health by emphasizing the importance of an active lifestyle.

Subscription services that deliver healthy snacks or meal kits can be a real time-saver for busy families and provide opportunities to introduce variety into a child's diet without the hassle of meal planning and grocery shopping every week.

Schools play a pivotal role in a child's nutrition, and it can be advantageous to have a dialogue with school administrators about their cafeteria offerings. Familiarize yourself with available resources to advocate for healthier options within the school environment.

Finally, consistent education is the backbone of sustaining healthy eating habits. There's an abundance of literature—books, scientific journals, and periodicals dedicated to nutrition and child health. Diving into these can equip you with the latest research and methodologies for continued learning.

With these resources and tools at your disposal, you'll be better positioned to foster an environment that supports healthy eating and contributes to the overall well-being of the children in your care. Remember, the journey towards a healthier lifestyle is always evolving, and staying informed and equipped will make all the difference.

Glossary of Nutritional Terms

Navigating the world of child nutrition can sometimes feel like learning a new language. With so many terms and concepts, it's crucial to have a solid grasp of the basics. This glossary will get you on a first-name basis with the nutritional terms essential in fostering healthful eating habits in children. Let's shape a brighter and healthier future, one word at a time!

Macronutrients

Carbohydrates: A major food group that's a primary source of energy for kids. They're found in foods like fruits, vegetables, bread, and pasta.

Proteins: The building blocks of muscles and tissues. Proteins are necessary for growth and repair and are found in meat, dairy, nuts, and legumes.

Fats: An essential nutrient that supports cell growth, brain development, and overall health. Healthy fats are found in foods such as avocados, nuts, and fish.

Vitamins and Minerals

Vitamins: Organic compounds that are vital for normal growth, metabolism, and good health. Examples include vitamin C, found in oranges, and vitamin D, obtained from sunlight exposure.

Minerals: Inorganic elements that help build strong bones, make hormones, and regulate the heartbeat, among other functions. Calcium and iron are common minerals.

Micronutrients

Essential vitamins and minerals that the body requires in small quantities. Despite their size, they pack a significant punch in terms of health benefits.

Food Allergies and Intolerances

Food Allergy: An immune system reaction that occurs soon after eating a certain food, even in small amounts.

Food Intolerance: Difficulty in digesting certain foods, which can cause unpleasant gastrointestinal symptoms.

Hydration

Water: The most essential nutrient for life. Adequate hydration is vital for all bodily functions, especially for growing children.

Dietary Restrictions

Specific limitations on a person's diet, which can be due to allergies, intolerances, or personal choices, such as following a vegetarian or vegan diet.

Whole Foods

Minimally processed foods that are closer to their natural state, offering a wealth of nutrients. Think fresh fruits, vegetables, grains, meats, and dairy.

Processed Snacks

Food items that have been significantly modified from their original form, often with added sugar, salt, and preservatives, which are not ideal for everyday consumption.

Sustainable Eating

An approach to food that considers nutrition and the environmental impact, with a focus on seasonal, locally-sourced, and minimally processed foods.

Understanding these terms is like having your very own nutrition compass. They'll guide you in making informed choices that nurture the well-being of children in your care. By speaking the language of nutrition fluently, you'll foster healthy habits that kids can carry into adulthood. Let's embark on the journey to better health with confidence and clarity!